Yoga-Sūtras of Patañjali, Made Easy

पातञ्जलयोगदर्शनदीपिका

Body Mind & Soul

Prof. Ratnakar Narale

Ratnakar
PUSTAK BHARATI
BOOKS-INDIA

Author :

Dr. Ratnakar Narale

B.Sc. (Nagpur), M.Sc. (Pune), Ph.D. (IIT), Ph.D. (Kalidas Sanskrit Univ.);

Prof. Hindi. Ryerson University, Toronto.

web : www.books-india.com * email : books.india.books@gmail.com

Book Title :

Yoga Sutras of Patanjali, Made Easy. पातञ्जलयोगदर्शनदीपिका ।

Published by :

PUSTAK BHARATI (Books-India)

Division of PC PLUS Ltd.

For :

Sanskrit Hindi Research Institute, Toronto

ISBN 978-1-897416-53-23

ISBN 978-1-897416-53-2

90000

9 781897 416532

Dedicated to

My Caring Wife
Sunita Ratnakar Narale
and my Loving Grandchildren
Samay Narale
Sahas Narale
Saanjh Narale
Saaya Narale

MAIN INDEX

INTRODUCTION

योगेन चित्तस्य पदेन वाचां मलं शरीरस्य च वैद्यकेन ।
योऽपाकरोत्तं प्रवरं मुनीनां पतञ्जलिं प्राञ्जलिरानतोस्मि ।

(For the purification of heart, speech and and body,
I bow to Patañjali, the supreme sage, the giver of body-science.)

Sanskrit is an ornate and poetic language. The immortal verses of its rich literature are composed by the ancient sages in *shlokas, sūtras* an *mantras.* The best examples of the vast *shloka*-literature are the epics of *Rāmāyaṇa* of Vālmīki and *Mahābhārata* of Vyāsa. Similarly, the preeminent examples of *sūtra*-literature are the *brahma-sūtras* of Bādrāyaṇa and *yoga-sūtras* of Patañjali and the most common examples of the *mantras* are *bij mantras, mūla mantras* and *siddhi mantras.*

The m∘ word *'śloka'* comes from verb root √*ślok* (भ्वादि∘ आत्मने∘ सक∘ √श्लोक् + अच्) to praise, to compose in verse, The *shlokas* are written in *anuṣṭubh* meter, according to the rules given in the following *shloka.*

'श्लोके' षष्ठं सदा दीर्घं लघु च पञ्चमं तथा ।
अक्षरं सप्तमं दीर्घं तृतीये प्रथमे पदे । ।

(In a *śloka*, there are four quartets *(pāda)*, each with eight syllables.
The fifth syllable of each quarter should be short,
the sixth long and the seventh alternately long and short in the odd and even quarters).

The n∘ word *'sūtra'* comes from the verb root √*sūtr* (चुरादि∘ परस्मै∘ सक∘ √सूत्र् + अच्) to string, to thread together, to formulate, to equate, to write in short rule, to systematize. The *sūtras* are not composed in any meter, but are written in minimum words according to the rules given in the following *shloka.*

अल्पाक्षरमसंदिग्धं सारवद्विश्वतोमुखम् ।
अस्तोभमनवद्यं च सूत्रं सूत्रविदो विदुः । ।

(A formula written in minimum words, without any confusion,

which includes the complete summary of the thought,
which can not be criticized and which is all encompassing, is called *sūtra,* by the *sūtra*-knowers)

The n∘ word *'mantra'* comes from the verb root √*mantr* (चुरादि॰ आत्मने॰ सक॰ √मन्त्र् + अच् *or* घञ्) to deliberate, to take counsel. A *mantra* are not written as a meaningful verse, but it is simply a series of characters, each of which may not have a meaning, but if uttered in a proper string (even the *mantras* which are to be whispered in ear), they have a secret power of achieving a desired fruit by arousing the inner energy of the receiver.

मकारो मननं प्राह त्रकारस्त्राणमुच्यते ।
मननत्राणसंयुक्तो मन्त्रमित्यभीधीयते ।।

(The character 'm' in the *man* (मन:) is meditation, character 'tr' in *trāṇ* (त्राणं) is protection, together they form a *mantra* which is rightly called a union of concentration and protection)

Therefore, these *yoga-sūtras* are the formulas written in least possible words to render an all-inclusive summary of Patañjali's teachings. In order to understand a *sūtra,* the reader (or the translator) must be able to fill in the appropriate connecting words or phrases, to evolve the condensed formula into a detailed thought. I have made every effort to evolve each *yoga-sūtra* first into Sanskrit and English phrases and then, using the same words, into English sentences. I hope, this way, the readers will be able to learn *Patañjali's yoga-ṣtras* with ease.

पातञ्जलमहाभाष्यचरकप्रतिसंस्कृतैः ।
मनोवाक्कायदोषाणां हन्त्रेऽहिपतये नमः ।।

(I slute Patañjali, the remover of faults from my mind, speech and body
by his *yoga-sūtras*)

Ratnakar

THE DEFINITIONS EMBEDED IN THE YOGA SUTRAS

1.1 अथ योगानुशासनम् । *Atha yogānuśāsanam*

* The Successive Tradition of the Discipline is called *'yoga'*

1.2 योगश्चित्तवृत्तिनिरोधः । *yogaś-citta-vṛtti-nirodhaḥ*

* This Discipline or State of Restraint of thought is called as *'yoga'*

1.3 यदा द्रष्टुः स्वरूपेऽवस्थानम् । *yadā draṣṭuḥ sva-rūpe-'vasthānam*

* When the State of Restraint of Thought of the *yogī* is attained, that Stable State is also called as *'yoga'*

1.7 प्रत्यक्षानुमानागमाः प्रमाणानि । *pratyakṣ-ānumān-āgamāḥ*

* Those which are cognizable conjectures, as well as the precepts of the *veda*, are called *pramāṇas* (proofs, standards).

1.8 विपर्ययो मिथ्याज्ञानमतद्रूपप्रतिष्ठम् । *viparyayo mithyājñānam-a-tadrupa-pratiṣṭham*

* The False Inference, which is not present in the true nature, is called as *'viparyayaḥ'* (perversion).

1.9 शब्दज्ञानानुपाती वस्तुशून्यो विकल्पः । *śabda-jñānānupātī vastu-śūnyo vikalpaḥ*

* That understanding which is obtained by hearing, that perception, devoid of substance, is called as *'vikalpaḥ.'*

1.10 अभावप्रत्ययालम्बना वृत्तिर्निद्रा । *a-bhāva-pratyayālambanā vṛttir-nidrā*

* The state of mind, which is achieved through the conviction that is based on absence of observation, is called as *'nidrā'* (slumber).

1.11 अनुभूतविषयासम्प्रमोषः स्मृतिः । *anubhūta-viṣayāsampramoṣaḥ smṛtiḥ*

* The experience attained through the revelation of the subject of the five mind-sets is called as *'smṛtiḥ'* (revelation).

1.13 तत्र स्थितौ यत्नोऽभ्यासः । *tatra sthitau yatno-'bhyāsaḥ*

* The effort made for the training practice and abstinence of the mind is called as *'abhyāsaḥ'* (practice).

1.15 दृष्टानुश्राविकविषयवितृष्णस्य वशीकारसंज्ञा वैराग्यम् । *dṛṣṭānuśrāvika-viṣaya-vitṛṇasya vaśikāra-sañjñā vairāgyam*

* That state of the *yogī*, the subject of which is witnessed and heard, and of which there is no desire or attachment, that state is called as *'vashikāraḥ,'* that alone is to be also known as *'vairagyam'* (non-attachment).

1.16 तत्परं पुरुषख्यातेर्गुण–वैतृष्ण्यम् । *tat-param puruṣa-khyāter-guṇa-vaitṛṣṇyam*

* When the *yogī* has no desire for attributes such as form, taste, smell, touch, etc., then that absence of the desire for the subjects of passions is called as *'para-vairāgyam.'*

1.17 वितर्कविचारानन्दास्मितानुगमात्सम्प्रज्ञातः । *vitarka-vićārānandāsmitānugāmāt-samprajñātaḥ*

* From the conformity of reflection, of contemplation, of bliss and of indifference, the *yoga* of the *yogī* is called as *'samprajñātaḥ.'*

1.18 विरामप्रत्ययाभ्यासपूर्वः संस्कारशेषोऽन्यः । *virāma-pratyayābhyāsa-pūrvaḥ saṁskāra-śeṣo-'nyaḥ*

* The cessation of conviction, of which the previous state is practice, and in which only previous impression on mind remains, that *yoga* is called as *'anyaḥ.'*

1.19 भवप्रत्ययो विदेहप्रकृतिलयानाम् । *bhavapratyayo videha-prakṛti-layānām*

* Of them by whom study of coming out from the bondage of the body as well as the practice of attaining the original pure state of their nature is attained, their *yoga* is called as *'bhavapratyayaḥ.'*

1.24 क्लेशकर्मविपाकाशयैरपरामृष्टः पुरुषविशेष ईश्वरः । *kleśa-karma-vipākāśayair-aprāmarṣṭaḥ puruṣa-viśeṣa īśvaraḥ from full devotion*

* He who is not afflicted by perversion of mind, by insensitivity, by attachment, by affliction, by hatred and by fear of death; and by *karma*, and by desire in the fruit of *karma*, and by a combination of these, that supreme person is called *'īśvaraḥ.'*

1.25 तत्र निरतिशयं सर्वज्ञबीजम् । *tatra nir-atiśatam sarva-bījam*

* He, from whom and in whom all knowledge originates and culminates and than whom nothing excels, to that supreme person they call *'niratiśayaḥ.'*

1.42 तत्र शब्दार्थज्ञानविकल्पैः सङ्कीर्णा सवितर्का समापत्तिः । *tatra śabdārtha-jñāna-vikalpaiḥ saṅkīrṇā sa-vitarkā samāpattiḥ*

* That state of 'oneness' of mind, equipped with senses such as hearing, objects such as purpose, and contrivances as perception, is known as *'savitarkā' (tainted) samādhi.*

1.43 स्मृतिपरिशुद्धौ स्वरूपशून्येवार्थमात्रनिर्भासा निर्वितर्का । *smṛti-pari-śuddhau svarūpa-śūnye-vārtha-mātra-nirbhāsā nir-vitarkā*

* When the aspects such as hearing and conviction are not in the reminiscence, such emptied pure in the original form and one pointed state of mind is called as *'nirvitarkā samādhi'* (untainted *samādhi*)

1.44 एतयैव सविचारा निर्विचारा च सूक्ष्मविषया व्याख्याता । *eta-yaiva sa-vićārā nir-vićārā ća sūkṣma-viṣayā vyākhyātā*

* The *samādhi* previously described with the names as *'savitarkā'* and *'nirvitarkā'* relating to the subtle aspects, are also known as *'savichārā,'* i.e. *samādhi* with discrimination and *'nirvichārā'* i.e. *samādhi* without discrimination,

1.46 ता एव सबीजः समाधिः । *tā eva sa-bīja samādhiḥ*

* The group of all these *samādhis* is collectively calles as *'sabīja-samādhi'* i.e. *samādhi* with a common element.

1.48 ऋतम्भरा तत्र प्रज्ञा । *ṛtambharā tatra prajñā*

* In that *samādhi,* the mind of the *yogī* is known as *ṛtambharā'* i.e. faithful.

1.51 तस्यापि निरोधे सर्वनिरोधान्निर्बिज: समाधि: । *tasyāpi nirodhe sarva-nirodhānnir-bījaḥ samādhiḥ*

* On prohibiting the impression of the *ṛtambharā* thinking also, as a result of prohibition of all influences, that *samādhi,* without any source of influence, is called as *nirbīja-samādhi.* i.e. *samādhi* without a common element.

2.1 तप: स्वाध्यायेश्वरप्रणिधानानि क्रियायोग: । *tapaḥ svādhyāye-śvara-praṇidhāni kriyāyogaḥ*

* The discipline of (i) austerity of performing righteous actions according to one's own inborn nature, (ii) study of scriptures and (iii) devotion to God is called as *'kriyā-yoga.'*

2.5 अनित्याशुचिदु:खानात्मसु नित्यशुचिसुखात्मरविद्या । *anityāśuchi-duḥkhānātmasu nitya-śuci-sukhātmar-avidyā*

* The perception of permanence in impermanent, righteousness in unrighteous, happiness in suffering and manifest in the unmanifest, is called as *'avidyā* (influenced of mind). '

2.6 दृग्दर्शनशक्त्योरेकात्मतेवास्मिता । *dṛg-darśana-śaktyo-'rekātmatevāsmitā*

* The illusion of indifference between life-principle and material-principle is called as *'asmitā.'* (illusion of indifference).

2.7 सुखानुशयी राग: । *sukhānuśayī rāgaḥ*

* The attachment, situated behind the conviction of happiness, is called as *'rāga.'* (attachment)

2.8 दु:खानुशयी द्वेष: । *duḥkhānuśayī dveṣaḥ*

* The hatred situated behind the affliction of pain is called as *'dveṣaḥ.'* (hatred)

2.9 स्वरसवाही विदुषोऽपि तथारूढोऽभिनिवेश: । *sva-rasa-vāhī viduṣo-'pi tatha-rūḍho-bhiniveśaḥ*

* The inherent affliction of fear of death that exists in wise people also, is called as *'abhiniveśaḥ.'*

2.18 प्रकाशक्रियास्थितिशीलं भूतेन्द्रियात्मकं भोगापवर्गार्थं दृश्यम् । *prakāśa-kriyāsthiti-śīlam bhūte-ndriyatmakam bhogāpavargārtham dṛśyam*

* That, of which nature is *sat-guṇaḥ, rajo-guṇaḥ* and *tamo-guṇaḥ* and the beings with their eleven organs of which the purpose is experience and which has visible nature, that is called as *'dṛśyam.'*

2.20 द्रष्टा दृशिमात्र: शुद्धोऽपि प्रत्ययानुपश्य: । *draṣṭā dṛśimātraḥ śuddho'pi pratyānupaśyaḥ*

* The life principle that is called *atmā,* even though eternal, by his association with cognition he behaves accordingly, and therefore, he is called as *'dṛṣṭā'* (beholder).

2.23 स्वस्वामिशक्त्यो: स्वरूपोपलब्धिहेतु: संयोग: । *sva-svāmi-śaktyoḥ sva-rūpo-palabdhi-hetuḥ saṁyogaḥ*

* Coming together of the purpose of your physical principle and the *ātmā* is called as *'saṁyogaḥ'* (union).

2.25 तदभावात्संयोगाभावो हानं तद्दृशेः कैवल्यम् । *tad-abhāvāt-saṁyogābhavo hānam taddṛśeḥ kaivalyam*

* With the absence of that perversion of mind, *saṁyoga* does not take place. And from that, non-existence of future pains also occurs. Therefore, that not coming together of the living principle *ātmā* (with your physical principle), is called as *'kaivalyam'* (liberation)

2.26 विवेकख्यातिरविप्लवा हानोपायः । *viveka-khyātir-aviplavā hanopāyaḥ*

* That untrained, of which the designation is *'vivekaḥ,'* (discernment), should also be understood as comprehension.

2.27 तस्य सप्तधा प्रान्तभूमिः प्रज्ञा । *tasyasaptadhā prānta-bhūmiḥ prajñā*

* That discernment, by which sevenfold aura is achieved, is called as *'prajñā'* (cognition).

2.29 यमनियमासनप्राणायामप्रत्याहारधारणाध्यानसमाधयोऽष्टावङ्गानि ।

yama-niyamāsana-prāṇāyāma-partyāhāra-dhāraṇādhyāna-samādhayo-'ṣṭāv-aṅgāni

* (i) Self control, (ii) observance, (iii) posture, (iv) breath control, (v) withholding, (vi) focus on aim (vii) concentration and (viii) meditation are called *'aṣta-yogāṅgāni'* (eight components) of *yoga.*

2.30 अहिंसासत्यास्तेयब्रह्मचर्यापरिग्रहाः यमाः । *ahiṁsāsatyāsteya-brahmacharyāparigrahāḥ yamāḥ*

* (i) Non-violence through deeds, words and thought by forsaking of all forms of killing, harm, treachery and enmity, (ii) truthfulness, (iii) non-stealing, (iv) sexual restraint and (v) non-hoarding are called as *'pañća-amāḥ'* (five self-controls) .

2.32 शौचसन्तोषतपःस्वाध्यायेश्वरप्रणिधानि नियमा । *sauća-santoṣa-tapaḥ-svādhyāye-śvara-praṇidhāni niyamāḥ*

* Purity, contentment, austerity, study of scriptures and faith in God are called as five *'niyamāḥ,'* (observances).

2.34 वितर्का हिंसादयः कृतकारिताअनुमोदिता लोभक्रोधमोहपूर्वका मृदुमध्याधिकमात्रा दुःखाज्ञानानन्तफला इति प्रतिपक्षभावम् । *vitarkā hiṁsādayaḥ kṛta-kāritāanumoditā lobha-krodha-moha-pūrvakā mṛdu-madhyādhika-mātrā duḥkhājñānā-nanta-phalā iti prati-pakṣa-bhāvam*

* The hindering emotions to self control and observances such as violence etc. which are of three types, namely self created, induced by others and instigated by others. Of these three types of sentiments, some are minor, some are moderate and some are of severe influence. They all give endless anguish and perversion in the form of a result. These are to be considered as *'doṣāḥ'* (obstacles).

2.46 स्थिरसुखमासनम् । *sthira-sukham-āsanam*

* The Steady State attained with ease is called as *'āsanam.'*

2.49 तस्मिन्सति श्वासप्रश्वासयोर्गतिविच्छेदः प्राणायामः । *tasmin-sati śsāsa-praśvāsayor-gati-vićchedaḥ prāṇāyāmaḥ*

* In the success of the *āsanam* of the *siddhiḥ,* the control of the rate of the in-breath and of out-breath is called as *'prāṇāyāmaḥ.'*

2.51 बाह्याभ्यन्तरविषयाक्षेपी चतुर्थः । *bāhyābhyantara-viṣayākṣepī ćturthaḥ*

* By keeping away the external and the internal thoughts, the *prāṇāyamaḥ* that occurs automatically is called *'ćaturthaḥ,'* (the fourth) *prāṇāyamaḥ.*

2.54 स्वविषयसम्प्रयोगे चित्तस्वरूपानुकार इवेन्द्रियाणां प्रत्याहारः । *sva-viṣaya-samprayoge ćitta-svarūpānukāra ive-ndriyān,ām pratyāhāraḥ*

* Becoming of the nature of sense organs analogous to one's own original inborn nature, by keeping away the internal and external thoughts, is called as *'pratyāhāraḥ'* (conditioning).

3.1 देशबन्धश्चित्तस्य धारणा । *deśa-bandha-śćittasya dhāraṇā*

* Stabilizing of mind in place is called as *'dhāraṇā'* (steady abstraction of mind)

3.2 तत्र प्रत्ययैकतानता ध्यानम् । *tatra pratyai-ktānatā dhyānam*

* Outside or inside the body, wherever the mind stays in steady abstraction, the one-pointedness of the absorption is called as *'dhyānam'* (concentration).

3.3 तदेवार्थमात्रनिर्भासं स्वरूपशून्यत्वमिव समाधिः । *tad-evā̃-rtha-mātra-nirbhāsam svarūpa-śūnyatvam-iva samādhiḥ*

* While concentrating, when only the perception of the aim remains and the own nature of mind becomes like vacuum, then that state is called as *'samādhiḥ'* (meditation).

3.4 त्रयमेकत्रम् संयमः । *trayam-ekatram sam̃yamaḥ*

* When the steady abstraction, concentration and meditation exist in one goal, then that trio of goals is called as *'sam̃yamaḥ'* (restraint).

3.9 व्युत्थाननिरोधसंस्कारयोरभिभवप्रादुर्भावौ निरोधक्षणचित्तान्वयो निरोधपरिणामः ।
vyutthāna-nirodha-sam̃skārayor-abhibhava-prādurbhāvau nirodha-kṣaṇa-ćittānvayo nirodha-pariṇāmaḥ

* In the two states namely, hinderence and dissolution of the impression on the mind, and of the two states namely, appearance and upsurge of the impression on the mind, at the time of hinderence, the control of mind becoming according to impressions on mind is called as the *'nirodha pariṇāmaḥ'* (consequence of restraint).

3.10 तस्य प्रशान्तवाहिता संस्कारात् । *tasya praśāntavāhitā sam̃skārāt*

* From that diminished impression on mind, the tranquil flowing state of mind is called as *'praśāntavāhitā'* (calmly streaming state).

3.11 सर्वार्थतैकाग्रतयोः क्षयोदयौ चित्तस्य समाधिपरिणामः । *sarvārthaikāgratayoḥ kṣayo-dayau ćittasya samādhi-pariṇāmaḥ*

* The two way diminution of all matters in the state of one-pointedness of mind and increase in the state of one-pointedness of mind in any one matter is called as *'samādhi-pariṇāmaḥ'* (consequence of meditation) .

3.12 ततः पुनः शान्तोदितौ तुल्यप्रत्ययौ चित्तस्यैकाग्रतापरिणामः । *tataḥ punaḥ śānto-ditau tulya-pratyayau cittasyai-kāgratāpariṇāmaḥ*

* Thereafter, when tranquility and unrest both come to an equilibrium, then that state of mind is called as *'ekāgratā-pariṇāmaḥ'* (consequence of one-pointedness).

3.14 शान्तोदिताव्यपदेश्यधर्मानुपाति धर्मी । *śānto-ditāvyapadeśya-dharmānupāti dharmī*

* The virtue that is present in the past, present and future attitude, is called as *'dharmī'* (righteous).

3.43 बहिरकल्पिता वृत्तिर्महाविदेहा ततः प्रकाशावरणक्षयः । *bhir-kalpitā vṛttir-mahāvidehā tataḥ prakāśāvaraṇa-kṣayaḥ*

* The natural state outside the body is called as *'mahā-videhaḥ'*

4.1 जन्मौषधिमन्त्रतपःसमाधिजाः सिद्धयः । *janmauṣadhi-mantra-tapaḥ-samādhihāḥ siddhayaḥ*

* Borne out of birth, borne out of a remedy, borne out incantation, borne out of austerity and borne out of meditation, are five *siddhis* (successes).

4.33 क्षणप्रतियोगी परिणामापरान्तनिर्ग्राह्यः क्रमः । *kṣaṇa-pratiyogī pariṇāmāparānta-nir-grāhyaḥ kramaḥ*

* At each moment sequentially, a transient thing, of which nature of fruit becomes clear at the end, that process is called as *'kramaḥ'* (sequential perception).

4.34 पुरुषार्थशून्यानां गुणानां प्रतिप्रसवः कैवल्यं स्वरूपप्रतिष्ठा वा चितिशक्तेरिति । *puruṣārtha-sūnyānām guṇānām pratiprasavaḥ kaivalyam svarūpa-pratiṣṭhā vā citi-śakter-iti*

* Those who have completed the four basic stages of human life and come to a zero state, return of their *gunas* to original state is '*kaivalyam*' (liberation), or return of the sway of the *ātmā* to its original point, is *kaivalya* thus one should understand.

4.34 पुरुषार्थशून्यानां गुणानां प्रतिप्रसवः कैवल्यं स्वरूपप्रतिष्ठा वा चितिशक्तेरिति । *puruṣārtha-sūnyānām guṇānām pratiprasavaḥ kaivalyam svarūpa-pratiṣṭhā vā citi-śakter-iti*

* Those who have completed the four basic stages of human life and come to a zero state, return of their *gunas* to original state is '*kaivalyam*' (liberation), or return of the sway of the *ātmā* to its original point, is *kaivalya* thus one should understand.

साम्येन वासनात्यागं मनसा देहनिग्रहम् ।
चित्तवृत्तेर्निरोधं तं ब्रूते योगं पतञ्जलिः ।।

(रत्नाकरः)

Yoga-Sūtras of Patañjali

पातञ्जलयोगदर्शनम् ।

Pātañjalayogadarṣhanam

1. समाधिपादः ।

Samādhipādaḥ

योगानुशासनम् ।

yogānushasanam

The Science of Yoga

1.1 अथ योगानुशासनम् । (अथ योग–अनु–शासनम् ।)

Atha yogānuśāsanam *(Atha yoga-anu-śāsanam)*

(i) अथ *atha* = अथ प्रारभ्यते *atha prārabhyate* = here begins

(ii) योगानुशासनम् *yoga-anu-śāsanam* = योग–विषयस्य अनुशासनम्, परम्परागतं योगशास्त्रम्

paramparāgatam yogashāstram = **the successive tradition of the discipline** called "yoga."

(iii) योग *yoga* = Yoga

(iv) अनुशासनम् *anu-śāsanam* = discipline.

NOTE : for the **Easy Learning** of the Sutras, PLEASE read all the ✍ **Comments**

📖 Here begins the Successive Tradition of the Discipline called *'yoga.'*

✍ **Comments :** Maharshi Patañjali says, Yoga is the "discipline" that has come down to us through the "Teacher-disciple tradition" from the ancient times.

As the Bhagavad-Gita says in Chapter iv : Lord Krishna told the Yoga first to Manu Vivasvān, Vivasvān told it to his son disciple Vaivasvān, Vivasvān to his son Ikṣavāku, Ikṣavāku to his disciple royal sages, the royal sages to mahā-rishis, the mahārishis to their disciple rishis, rishis to the *yogī*-students, and so on, came to us.

योगः ।

Yogaḥ

1. Yoga Defined

1.2 योगश्चित्तवृत्तिनिरोधः । (योगः चित्त-वृत्ति-निरोधः ।)

yogaścittavṛttinirodhaḥ (yogaḥ-ćitta-vṛtti-nirodhaḥ)

(i) योगः *'yoga'* = एतत् शास्त्रम् **this discipline** called yoga

(o) चित्त-वृत्ति-निरोधः *ćitta-vṛtti-nirodhaḥ* =

(i) चित्तवृत्तेः (चित्तम् *chittam* = mind); (वृत्तिः *vṛttiḥ* = mind-set)

ćittasya = चित्तस्य, चेतसः, मनसः, अन्तःकरणस्य, हृदयस्य, विचारस्य of state mind, of heart, of thought

vṛtteḥ = वृत्तेः, अवस्थायाः, प्रकृतेः of the attitude, = **the state of restrained mind set.**

(iii) निरोधः *nirodhaḥ* = निग्रहः, अवरोधः, प्रतिबन्धः, प्रतिरोधः restraint

(iv) 'योगः' 'yoga' = योगः इति उच्यते *yogaḥ iti uchyate* = is called as **'yoga'**

📖 This Discipline or the State of "Restraint of mind-set" is called as *'yoga.'*

✍ **Comments :** Then Patañjali, further tells us that : the Discipline of "Restraint of mind-set" is *yoga.* And the body condition with which this restraint (focus of mind) is achieved is called "*Asana.*" The process of attaining the right body posture and restraint of thought is *Sadhanā.* The success is "*Siddhi.*" The restraint of thought is "*Dhyānam* or *Samādhi*" (Contemplation or Meditation). Remember, *samādhi* is not so called "thinking of nothing," because "nothing" is also a thing. A 'thing' is the object of Meditation. How to choose the right object for the meditation for the desired success, is explained by Patañjali in Chapter 3.

1.3 तदा द्रष्टुः स्वरूपेऽवस्थानम् । (तदा द्रष्टुः स्व-रूपे अव-स्थानम् ।)

tadā draṣṭuḥ svarūpe'vasthānam (*tadā draṣṭuḥ sva-rūpe ava-sthānam*)

(i) तदा *tadā* = यदा चित्तस्य वृत्तेः निरोधः भवति तदा when the **state of restrained mind set** is attained, then

(ii) द्रष्टुः *draṣṭuḥ* = पश्यतः, योगिनः of the yogī

(iii) स्वरूपे *sva-rūpe* = स्व-रूपे, स्वस्य भावे, आत्मनि, स्व-प्रकृतौ **in one's own self**

(iv) अवस्थानम् *ava-sthānam* = सा स्थिरा स्थितिः **that stable state**

(v) अपि 'योगः' इति उच्यते *'api yogaḥ' iti uchyate* = is also called as 'yoga'

When the State of Restraint of Mind-Set in one's own self is attained, that Stable State of the yogi is also called as *'yoga.'*

Comments : When one achieves success (siddhi) in the restraint of thought, that "stable state" of success in the discipline, is also called Yoga. Remember, here the word "stable" is important.

1.4 वृत्तिसारूप्यमितरत्र । (वृत्ति-सा-रूप्यम् इतरत्र ।)

vṛttisārūpyamitartra (*vṛtti-sā-rūpyam itartra*)

(i) इतरत्र *itartra* = अन्ये समये at other times, when his mind is not in the stable state and restrained on one focus.

(ii) योगिनः *yoginaḥ* = of the yogī

(o) वृत्तिसारूप्यम् *vṛtti-sā-rūpyam* =

(iii) वृत्तेः *vṛtteḥ* = अवस्थायाः, स्थितेः, स्व-रूपस्य of the state, of the mind-set

(iv) सारूप्यम् *sā-rūpyam* = तस्य स्वभाव:, मूल-वृत्ते:, प्रकृते: of normal nature

(iv) इव भवति *it bhavati* = is like, is similar to, becomes equal to

📖 **At other times, when his mind is not in the stable state and restrained on one focus, the state of the *yogī* is like his normal nature.**

✍ **Comments :** A *yogi* whose mind is not in engaged in contemplation of any one object of meditation, the *yogi* is not in the state of *yoga*. He is still a *yogi*, for he is a disciplined person.

वृत्ति: ।

Vṛttiḥ

2. Mind-set

1.5 वृत्तय: पञ्चतय्य: क्लिष्टाक्लिष्टा: । (वृत्तय: पञ्च-तय्य: क्लिष्टा: अक्लिष्टा: ।)

vṛttayaḥ pañćatayyaḥ kilṣṭākliṣṭāḥ (*vṛttayaḥ pañća-tayyaḥ kilṣṭāḥ a-kliṣṭāḥ*)

(i) वृत्तय: *vṛttayaḥ* = योगिन: वृत्तय: *yoginaḥ vṛttayaḥ* = योगिन: चित्तावस्था:, चित्तस्य अवस्था: the states of mind or **the mind-sets** of the yogī

(o) क्लिष्टाक्लिष्टा: *kilṣṭāḥ a-kliṣṭāḥ* =

(i) क्लिष्टा: *kilṣṭāḥ* = impaired

(ii) च *cha* = and

(iii) अक्लिष्टा: *a-kliṣṭāḥ* = non-impaired

(iv) च इति *cha iti* = thus

(v) पञ्चतय्य: *pañća-tayyaḥ* = पञ्च विधा: *pañća vidhāḥ* = **of five kinds**, of five types

(vi) वर्तन्ते *vartante* = are

📖 **The mind-sets of the *yogī* are of two kinds (i) impaired and (ii) non-impaired. Each of the two states has five kinds.**

✍ Comments : The mind sets of five types, in each of the two sets of mind, are shown in the following table :

वृत्तय: (Mind-sets)

1.	2.	3.	4.	5.
प्रमाणम् (Standard)	विपर्यय: (Error)	विकल्प: (Unreality)	निद्रा (Unawareness)	स्मृति: (Revelation)
i. लिष्टा (Impared)	i. लिष्टा (Impared)	i. लिष्टा (Impared)	i. लिष्टा (Impared)	i. लिष्टा (Impared)
ii. अश्लिष्टा (Unimpared)	ii. अश्लिष्टा (Unimpared)	ii. अश्लिष्टा (Unimpared)	ii. अश्लिष्टा (Unimpared)	ii. अश्लिष्टा (Unimpared)

1.6 प्रमाणविपर्ययविकल्पनिद्रास्मृतय: । (प्रमाण-विपर्यय-विकल्प-निद्रा-स्मृतय: ।)

pramāṇaviparyavikalpanidrāsmṛtayaḥ

(pramāṇa-viparya-vikalpa-nidrā-smṛtayaḥ)

(o) प्रमाण-विपर्यय-विकल्प-निद्रा-स्मृतय: *pramāṇa-viparya-vikalpa-nidrā-smṛtayaḥ* =

(i) प्रमाणम् pramāṇam = proof, something that is evident, apparent, obvious, tangible

(ii) विपर्यय: *viparyaḥ* = without proof, unclear, intangible, obscure

(iii) विकल्प: *vikalpaḥ* = indecision, uncertainty, doubt

(iv) निद्रा, सुप्ति: *nidrā* = languish, stupor, delusion, hallucination, trance

(v) च *cha* = and

(vi) 'स्मृतय:' *smṛtayaḥ* = the faculties of mind

(vii) इति मता: *iti matāḥ* = are considered as

📖 **Evident, non-evident, uncertainty, delusion and trance are considered as the five faculties of mind.**

✍ Comments : A thought in the mind could be based on (i) something that is manifest before him, such as a picture of a historic person; (ii) something that is non-visible to him, such as the historic person in the picture; (iii) something that is not for sure, such as "is this the really a picture of that historic person;" (iv) something that is a misconception, such as : one can talk to that historic person through the picture; (v) and a restful mind, without that picture before him, or without seeing that picture.

प्रमाणम् ।

Pramāṇam

3. Proof, Standard

1.7 प्रत्यक्षानुमानागमाः प्रमाणानि । (प्रत्यक्ष-अनुमान- आगमाः प्रमाणानि ।)

pratyakṣānumānāgamāḥ pramāṇāni *(pratyakṣa-anumāna-āgamāḥ pramāṇāni)*

(o) प्रत्यक्ष-अनुमान-आगमाः *pratyakṣa-anumāna-āgamāḥ* =

(i) प्रत्यक्षम् यत् *pratyakṣam yat* = दृगोचरम्, दृश्यम्, दृष्टम्, स्पष्टम् **that which is preceptible**, visible, present, cognizable

(ii) अनुमानम् *anumānam* = स-तर्कम्, अभ्यूहम्, ऊहम् conclusion, inference, guess, conjecture

(iii) आगमाः *āgamāḥ* = वेद-शास्त्र-विधानानि **precepts of the Veda,** precepts of the scriptures

(iv) ये *ye* = those which are

(v) ते 'प्रमाणानि' *te pramāṇāni* = तानि साक्ष्यानि, इयत्ताः, सिद्धयः those proofs

(vi) सन्ति *santi* = are

📖 **Those which are cognizable conjectures, as well as the precepts of the *veda*, are called the *pramāṇas* (proofs or the set standards).**

✍ Comments : The precepts of the *vaidic rishis*, put forth after generations of practical experiences, are regarded as the set-standards or the proofs, as good as the inferences of one's own practical knowledge is.

विपर्ययः ।

viparyayaḥ

4. Error

1.8 विपर्ययो मिथ्याज्ञानमतद्रूपप्रतिष्ठम् । (विपर्ययः मिथ्या-ज्ञानम् अतद्रूप-प्रतिष्ठम् ।)

viparyayo mithyājñānamatadrūpapratiṣṭham

(viparyayo mithyā-jñānam-a-tadrūpa-pratiṣṭham)

i) अ–तद्रुप–प्रतिष्ठम् *a-tadrūpa-pratiṣṭham* = यत् समक्षं नास्ति, यत् प्रत्यक्षं न विद्यते *yat pratyakṣham nāsti* = that which is not prsent

ii) अ–तद्रूपम् *a-tadrūpam* = तद् अ–रूपम्, सत्यम्, ऋतृम्, अयथार्थम्, अवितथम्, अकृत्रिमम् लक्षणम् that which is not the true nature

iii) प्रतिष्ठम् *pratiṣṭham* = विद्यमानम्, प्रत्यक्षम्, वर्तमानम्, उपस्थितम् present in

iv) तत् मिथ्या ज्ञानम् *tat mithya jñānam* = that false inference

v) 'विपर्यय:' *viparyayo* = मिथ्याज्ञानम् misunderstanding, mistake, error, misapprehension, perversion

vi) इति उच्यते *iti uchyate* = is known as, is called as

📖 **The False Inference, which is not present in the true nature, is called *'viparyayaḥ'* (error).**

✍ Comments : The erroneous or false inference which is away from the true fact, is a *viparyay.*

विकल्प: ।

vikalpaḥ

5. Unreality

1.9 शब्दज्ञानानुपाती वस्तुशून्यो विकल्प: । (शब्द-ज्ञान-अनुपाती वस्तु-शून्यो विकल्प: ।)

śabdajñānānupātī vastuśūnyo vikalpaḥ *(śabda-jñānāna-aupātī vastu-śūnyo vikalpaḥ)*

(o) शब्द–ज्ञान–अनुपाति *śabda-jñānā-aupātī* =

(i) अनुपातिन् (m. singular = *aupātī* अनुपाती) = the follower

(ii) ज्ञानम् *jñānānam* = प्रतीति:, बोध: understanding, perception, apprehension, conception, observation

(iii) यत् *yat* = that which is

(iv) शब्दैः *śabdaiḥ* = ध्वनिभिः, निनादैः through sounds, by hearing

(v) प्राप्यते *prāpyate* = अनुपद्यते, आयाति comes from, is obtained by

(vi) वस्तुशून्यः *vastu-śūnyaḥ* = अविद्यमानम् *a-vidyamānam* = अविषयकः विषयः devoid of substance

(vii) 'विकल्पः' *'vikalpaḥ'*

(viii) इति उच्यते *iti uchyate* = is known as, is called as

📖 **The follower of that understanding (i) which is obtained by hearing; or (ii) that perception, devoid of substance, is called as a *'vikalpaḥ'* (unreality).**

✍ Comments : The understanding based on something that is only heard or something that is devoid of a proof, is an unreality or a *vikalpa*.

निद्रावृत्तिः ।

nidrāvṛttiḥ

6. Unawareness

1.10 अभावप्रत्ययालम्बना वृत्तिर्निद्रा । (अ-भाव-प्रत्यय-आलम्बना वृत्तिः निद्रा ।)

abhāvapratyayālambanā vṛttir-nidrā

(a-bhāva-pratyaya-ālambanā vṛttir-nidrā)

(o) अभाव-प्रत्ययालम्बना *a-bhāva-pratyaya-ālambanā* =

(i) ज्ञानस्य *jñānasya* = of the understanding, perception, apprehension, conception, observation.

(ii) अभावस्य *a-bhāvasya* = अविद्यमानतायाः *a-vidyamānatāyāḥ* = of the bsence, non-presence

(iii) प्रतीतिम् *pratītim* = बोधम् the awareness

(iv) ग्रह्यमाणा *grahyamāṇā* = *feminine. adj.* which is achieved through

(v) आलंबना *ālambanā* = *f◦ noun.* the mental exercise

(vi) वृत्तिः *vṛttiḥ* = चित्तस्य अवस्था the state of mind

(vii) 'निद्रा' *'nidrā'* = unawareness

(viii) इति उच्यते *iti uchyate* = is known as, is called as

📖 **The state of mind, which is achieved through the mental exercise that is based on absence of (awareness and) perception, is called as *'nidrā'* (unawareness).**

✍ Comments : The unstable state of restful mind in which awareness of perception is not there, is *nidra*. Nidra does not necessarily mean the sleep or slumber, but it is the absence of awareness.

स्मृतिः ।

smṛtiḥ

7. Revelation

1.11 अनुभूतविषयासम्प्रमोषः स्मृतिः । (अनुभूत-विषय-असम्प्रमोषः स्मृतिः ।)

anubhūtaviṣayāsampramoṣaḥ smṛtiḥ

(anubhūta-viṣayā- aampramoṣaḥ smṛtiḥ)

(o) अनुभूत-विषय-असम्प्रमोषः *anubhūta-viṣayāsampramoṣaḥ* =

(i) अनुभूतस्य *anubhūtasya* = साक्षात् उपलब्धस्य, साकारस्य of the experience attained through the five mind-sets

(ii) विषयस्य *viṣayāsya* = प्रसङ्गस्य, व्यापारस्य, अर्थस्य of the subject

(iii) असम्प्रोषः *sampramoṣaḥ* = प्रकटनम्, आविर्भवनम्, प्रकाशनम् revelation

(iv) 'स्मृतिः' = *'smṛtiḥ'*

(v) इति उच्यते *iti uchyate* = is known as, is called as

📖 **The experience attained through the revelation of the subject of the (above mentioned) five mind-sets is called as *'smṛtiḥ'* (revelation).**

✍ Comments : The revelation of experience of mind set that is based on (i) something that is manifest, (ii) something that is non-visible; (iii) something that is not certain, (iv) something that is a misconception, and (v) and the mind in a trance : is a *smriti*.

1.12 अभ्यासवैराग्याभ्यां तन्निरोधः । (अभ्यास-वैराग्याभ्यां तन्-निरोधः ।)

abhyāsavairāgyābhyām tannirodhaḥ

(abhyāsa-vairāgyābhyām tan-nirodhaḥ)

(i) तत् *taṭ* = उपरोक्तस्य वृत्ति-पञ्चकस्य of the above mentioned five mind-sets

(ii) निरोधः *nirodhaḥ* = अवरोधः, प्रतिबन्धः, निग्रहः the restraint

(o) अभ्यास-वैराग्याभ्याम् *abhyāsa-vairāgyābhyām* =

(iii) अभ्यासेन *abhyāsena* = नित्यव्यवहारेण, नित्यवृत्त्या by regular training, by everyday performance

(iv) च *cha* = and

(v) वैराग्येण *vairāgyeṇa* = विरक्त्या, अनासक्त्या by non-attachment, by detachment, by abstinence

(vi) शक्यते *shakyate* = is possible

🕮 **The restraint of the above mentioned five mind-sets is possible by practice, regular training and by abstinence.**

✍ Comments : The control of the above mentioned five mind sets is possible through practice and abstinence. It has already been said in the Bhagavadgita (6:35 *abhyāsena vairāgyeṇa cha gṛhyate*), the yoga of control of mind is possible through *abhyasa* (practice) and *vairagya* (abstinence).

Please note that : in this book references are made to the quotes from the Bhagavad Gita, because the Gita (4.1) says : the first discourse on the Yoga was given by Lord Krishna to Vivasvan. Vivasvan then gave the yoga to Vaivasvan, then Vaisvan to Ikshavaku, Ikshvaku to the Royal sages, the sages to the Maharishis, the maharishis to the rishis, the rishis to their disciples, and so on and thus the yoga came to Patanjali and then it came down to us.

1.13 तत्र स्थितौ यत्नोऽभ्यासः । (तत्र स्थितौ यत्नः अभ्यासः ।)

tatra sthitau yatno'bhyāsaḥ *(tatra sthitau yatnaḥ abhyāsaḥ)*

(i) तत्र *tatra* = अभ्यास-वैराग्ययोः *abhyāsa vairāgyayaḥ* = in the training practice and abstinence

(ii) स्थितौ *sthitau* = चित्तस्य स्थिरतायै, मनसः दृढतायाम्, मनसः दृढतायै, चेतसः स्थायितायाम् in the or for the or of the mind

(iii) कृत: *kṛtaḥ* = done, made

(iv) यत्न: *yatnaḥ* = प्रयास:, चेष्टा, परिश्रम:, उपाय:, उद्योग: the effort

(v) 'अभ्यास:' 'abhyāsaḥ'

(vi) इति उच्यते *iti uchyate* = is known as, is called as

📖 **The effort that is made in the training and abstinence of the mind is called as *'abhyāsaḥ'* (practice).**

✍ Comments : As quoted above from the Gita (6:35), the control of mind and the training for abstinence, is called *abhyasa.*

1.14 स तु दीर्घकालनैरन्तर्यसत्काराऽऽसेवितो दृढभूमिः ।

(स तु दीर्घ–काल–नैरन्तर्य–सत्कार–आ–सेवितो दृढभूमिः ।)

sa tu dīrghakālanairantaryasatkārā"sevito dṛḍhabhumiḥ

(sa tu dīrgha-kāla-nairantarya-satkārā ā-sevito dṛḍha-bhumiḥ)

(i) तु *tu* = अपि च and, also

(ii) स: *saḥ* = स: अभ्यास: *saḥ abhyāsaḥ* = **that training practice**

(o) दीर्घ–काल–नैरन्तर्य–सत्कार–आ–सेवित: *dīrgha-kāla-nairantarya-satkārā ā-sevito dṛḍha-bhumiḥ* =

(iii) यदा *yadā* = when

(iv) दीर्घ *dīrgha* = आयत, अधिक long

(v) काल *kāla* = समय time

(vi) पर्यन्तम् *paryantam* = up to, for

(vii) निरन्तरम् *nirantaram* = अखण्डम्, सततम् non-stop

(viii) च *cha* = and

(ix) सत्कारपूर्वकं *satkāra-pūrvakam* = आदरपूर्वकम्, सम्मानपूर्वकम् with respect

(x) च क्रियते *cha kriyate* = is done

(o) दृढभूमि: *dṛḍha-bhumiḥ* =

(xi) तदा *tadā* = then

(xii) चित्तस्य अवस्था *chittasya avasthā* = **the state of mind**

(xiii) 'दृढभूमि' *dṛḍha-bhumiḥ* = स्थिरा *sthirā* = **steady**

(xiv) भवति *bhavati* = is, **becomes**, occurs, happens

📖 **And, when such practice is done for long time, non-stop and with respect, then the state of mind becomes steady.**

✍ Comments : With the self-control done for long time, steadily and with respect, the mind becomes steady. In the Gita (2:55) such *yogi* of steady mind is called *sthitaprajña.*

वैराग्यम् ।

vairāgyam

8. Non-attachment

1.15 दृष्टानुश्राविकविषयवितृष्णस्य वशीकारसंज्ञा वैराग्यम् ।

(दृष्ट-अनुश्राविक-विषय-वितृष्णस्य वशीकार-संज्ञा वैराग्यम् ।)

dṛṣṭānuśrāvikaviṣayavitṛṇasya vaśikārasañjñā vairāgyam

(dṛṣṭā-auśrāvika-viṣaya-vitṛṇasya vaśikāra-sañjñā vairāgyam)

(o) दृष्ट-अनुश्राविक-विषय-वितृष्णस्य *dṛṣṭā-auśrāvika-viṣaya-vitṛṇasya* =

(i) दृष्टस्य *dṛṣṭasya* = अवलोकितस्य, निरूपितस्य, लक्षितस्य, ईक्षितस्य of that which is witnessed

(ii) च *cha* = and

(iii) अनुश्राविकस्य *auśrāvikasya* = परम्परया श्रुतस्य, आकर्णितस्य, निशान्तस्य of that which is heard

(iv) विषयस्य *viṣayasya* = प्रकरणस्य, आस्वादस्य, व्यापारस्य of the subject

(v) वितृष्णस्य = विगततृष्णस्य, तृप्तस्य, सन्तुष्टस्य, कृतार्थस्य of which there is no desire or attachment

(vi) योगिनः *yoginaḥ* = of the yogī

(vii) वशीकार-संज्ञा *vashikāra-samjñā* = सा अवस्था, सा स्थितिः **that state**

(viii) 'वशीकार:' *'vashikāraḥ'*

(ix) इति उच्यते *iti uchyate* = is known as, is called as

(x) सा एव *sā eva* = that alone

(xi) 'वैराग्यम्' *'vairagyam'*

(xii) इति अपि मन्तव्या *iti api mantavyā* = is to be also known as

📖 **That state of the *yogī*, the subject of which is witnessed and heard, and of which there is no desire or attachment, that state is called as *'vashikāraḥ,'* that alone is to be also known as *'vairagyam'* (non-attachment).**

✍ Comments : The state of a yogi, in which the success is without the attachment and desire of the fruit, is called *vishikara*. In the Gita, this non-attachment is called *asakti* (13:9, 3:7) and the non-coveting for fruit is called *niṣkāma* or *nihspṛha* (2.71) .

1.16 तत्परं पुरुषख्यातेर्गुणवैतृष्ण्यम् ।

tatparam puruṣakhyāterguṇavaitṛṣṇyam

(tat-param puruṣa-khyāteḥ-guṇa-vaitṛṣṇyam)

(i) *guṇa-vaitṛṣṇyam* = गुण–वैतृष्ण्यम्, गुणानां, द्रव्यधर्माणाम्, रूपरसगन्धस्पर्शादयानाम् for attributes such as form, taste, smell, touch, etc.

(ii) तृष्णाया: *tṛṣṇāyāḥ* = कामनाया:, इच्छाया:, लालसाया: of the desire

(iii) अभाव: *abhāvaḥ* = अविद्यमानता absence

(iv) पुरुष–ख्याते *Puruṣa-khyāteḥ* = साधकस्य यदा वर्तते when the yogī has

(v) तदा *tadā* = then

(vi) तत् *tat* = तत् वैराग्यम्, विरक्ति:, अनासक्ति:, स: विषय–कामनाया: अभाव: that, that absence of the desire for the subjects of passions

(vii) परम् *param* = 'पर–वैराग्यम्' 'para-vairāgyam'

(viii) इति उच्यते *iti uchyate* = is known as, is called as

📖 **When the *yogī* has no desire for attributes such as form, taste, smell, touch, etc., then that absence of the desire for the subjects of passions is called as *'para-vairāgyam.'***

✍ Comments : The absence of passions or attachment is called *para-vairāgya.* In the Gita (2.56) it is called vita-rāga.

1.17 वितर्कविचारानन्दास्मितानुगमात्सम्प्रज्ञात: ।

vitarkavićārānandāsmitānugāmātsamprajñātaḥ

(vitarka-vićāra-ānanda-āsmitā-anugāmāt-samprajñātaḥ)

(o) वितर्क–विचार–आनन्द–अस्मिता–अनुगमात् *vitarka-vićārānandāsmitānugāmāt* =

(i) वितर्कस्य *vitarkasya* = ऊहापोहस्य, अनुमानस्य, सन्देहस्य from the conjecture, reflection

(ii) च *cha* = and

(iii) विचारस्य *vićārasya* = तर्कस्य, चिन्तनस्य, सङ्कल्पस्य of thought, of contemplation

(iv) च *cha* = and

(v) आनन्दस्य *ānandasya* = शान्ते:, प्रसन्नताया: of bliss, of elation

(vii) च *cha* = and

(vii) अस्मिताया: *asmitāyaḥ* = अभेदस्य of the indifference

(viii) च *cha* = and

(ix) अनुगमात् *anugāmāt* = संबन्धात्, चित्तवृत्ते: समाधानात् from the conformity

(x) सम्प्रज्ञात: *samprajñātaḥ* = योगिनो योग: 'सम्प्रज्ञात:' the yoga of the yogī is *samprajñātaḥ.*

(xi) इति उच्यते *iti uchyate* = is known as, is called as

📖 **From the conformity (i) of reflection, (ii) of contemplation, (iii) of bliss and (iv) of indifference, the *yoga* of the *yogī* is called as *'samprajñātaḥ.'***

✍ Comments : The samprajñata or the indifference with the other three attributes are collectively referred in the

Gita (6.9) as sama-buddhi, sama-bhuudi-yoga or the buddhiyoga.

1.18 विरामप्रत्ययाभ्यासपूर्वः संस्कारशेषोऽन्यः ।

virāmapratyayābhyāsapūrvaḥ saṁskāraśeṣo'nyaḥ

(virāma-pratyaya-ābhyāsa-pūrvaḥ saṁskāra-śeṣo-'nyaḥ)

(o) विराम–प्रत्यय–अभ्यास–पूर्वः *virāma-pratyaya-ābhyāsa-pūrvaḥ* =

(i) विरामः *virāmaḥ* = वृत्तिनिरोधस्य साधनम् the means of self control

(ii) प्रत्ययस्य *pratyayasya* = ज्ञानस्य of knowledge

(iii) अभ्यासः *ābhyāsaḥ* = नित्यप्रवृत्तिः, अभ्यसनम् practice

(iv) यस्य *yasya* = of which

(v) पूर्वः *pūrvaḥ* = प्राग्–अवस्था the previous state

(vi) भवति *bhavati* = is

(vii) संस्कार–शेषः *saṁskāra-śeṣaḥ* = यस्मिन् चित्तस्य स्वरूपं मात्र संस्कारः, मानसी शिक्षा एव in which only previous impression on mind

(viii) अवशिष्यते *avaśiṣyate* = remains

(ix) सः योगः *saḥ yogaḥ* = **that yoga**

(xii) 'अन्यः' **'anyaḥ'**

(xiii) इति उच्यते *iti uchyate* = **is called as**

📖 **With the means of self control, of which the previous state is the practice, and in which only the knowledge of previous impression on mind remains, that *yoga* is called *'anyaḥ.'***

✍ Comments : When with the practice of self control, only the pre-conviction impression remains in mind, then it is called *anya-yoga*. It is called *anya* because it is different from the other modes of yoga.

1.19 भवप्रत्ययो विदेहप्रकृतिलयानाम् ।

bhavapratyayo videhaprakṛtilayānām

(bhava-pratyayo videha-prakṛti-layānām)

(o) विदेह-प्रकृति-लयानाम् *videha-prakṛti-layānām* =

(ii) विदेह: *videhaḥ* = देहस्य बन्धनात् मुक्त्वा देहात् बहि: आगमनस्य अभ्यास: येषां दृढ: जात: तेषाम् of them by whom study of coming out from the bondage of the body is done

(iii) तथा च *tathā cha* = as well as

(iv) प्रकृति: *prakṛtiḥ* = मृत्यो: पूर्वं येषां साधना 'प्रकृतिलय-स्थितिम्' प्राप्ता भवति the practice of attaining the original pure state of their nature is attained

(v) तेषाम् *teṣām* = their

(vi) योग: yogaḥ

(vii) 'भवप्रत्यय:' *'bhavapratyayaḥ'*

(viii) इति उच्यते *iti uchyate* = is called as

📖 **Of them, by whom (i) the study of coming out from the bondage of the body (ii) as well as the practice of attaining the original pure state of their nature is attained, their yoga is called as *'bhavapratyayaḥ.'***

✍ Comments : When with extreme practice of the yoga, the yogi comes out the conformity of his body and experiences his original pure state, that yoga is *bhavapratya.*

1.20 श्रद्धावीर्यस्मृतिसमाधिप्रज्ञापूर्वक इतरेषाम् ।

śraddhāvīryasmṛtisamādhiprajñāpūrvaka itareṣām

(śraddhā-vīrya-smṛti-samādhi-prajñā-pūrvaka itareṣām)

(i) इतरेषाम् *itareṣām* = अन्येषां योगिनां योग: the yoga of other yogīs

(o) श्रद्धा-वीर्य-स्मृति-समाधि-प्रज्ञा-पूर्वक: *śraddhā-vīrya-smṛti-samādhi-prajñā-pūrvaka* =

(ii) श्रद्धा *śraddhā* = अविचला भावना, भक्तिपूर्णविश्वास: faith

(iii) तत्पश्चात् *tat-paśchāt* = followed by

(iv) वीर्यं *vīryam* = मनसः इन्द्रियाणां च सामर्थ्यम् strength of mind

(v) ततः *tataḥ* = then

(vi) स्मृतिः *smṛtiḥ* = पूर्व-संस्काराणां प्राकट्यम् revelation of previous impressions

(vii) तदनन्तरं *tad-nantaram* = and then

(viii) समाधिः *samādhiḥ* = समाहितस्य मनसः विषयेभ्यः विरक्तिः detachment

(ix) तदनु *tadanu* = तदा, तत्पश्चात्, ततः and then

(x) प्रज्ञा *prajñā* = बुद्धिः, ज्ञानम्, विचारः understanding, thought

(xi) पूर्वकः *pūrvakaḥ* = endowment with

(xii) इति क्रमेण *iti krameṇa* = in this order

(xiii) भवति *bhavati* = becomes

📖 **The *yoga* of other *yogīs* becomes in this order : (i) faith, followed by (ii) strength of mind, then (iii) revelation of previous impressions, and then (iv) their detachment and then (v) endowment with understanding.**

✍ Comments : The faith, strength of mind, revelation of previous impressions, detachment from those impressions and then understanding the yoga, are the five steps in the study of yoga and concentration of mind.

1.21 तीव्रसंवेगानामासन्नः ।

tīvrasam̐vegānāmāsannaḥ *(tīvra-sam̐vegānām-āsannaḥ)*

(i) तीव्र-संवेगानाम् *tīvra-sam̐vegānām* = येषां योगिनां अभ्यासस्य च वैराग्यस्य च साधनायाः संवेगः (गतिः) of those yogīs whose rate of success in practice of attainment and detachment

(ii) तीव्रा *tīvrā* = अत्यधिका, वेगवत्, शीघ्रा high, rapid

(iii) भवति *bhavati* = is

(iv) तेषाम् *teṣām* = for them

(v) आसन्नः *āsannaḥ* = सिद्धिः, साफल्यम्, कृतकार्यता, पूर्णता; समाधिः success in concentration of mind

(vi) अपि *api* = also

(vii) शीघ्रा *śighrā* = rapid

(viii) भवति *bhavati* = is

📖 **Of those *yogīs* whose rate of success in practice of attainment and detachment is rapid, for them successes in concentration of mind is also rapid.**

✍ Comments : When the above mentioned detachment is rapid, the success in concentration of mind is also rapid.

1.22 मृदुमध्याधिमात्रत्वात्ततोऽपि विशेषः ।

mṛdumadhyādhimātratvāttatao'pi viśeṣaḥ

(mṛdu-madhya-adhimātratvāt-tatao-'pi viśeṣaḥ)

(i) साधनायाः *sādhanāyaḥ* = of concentration of mind

(ii) वेगः *vegaḥ* = गतिः, मात्रा, मानम् the rate, speed

(o) मृदु-मध्य-अधिमात्रत्वात् *mṛdu-madhya-adhimātratvāt* =

(iii) मृदुः *mṛdu* = लघुः, मन्दः **slow**

(iv) मध्यः *madhyaḥ* = सामान्यः, साधारणः **moderate**;

(v) च *cha* = or, and

(vi) अधिमात्रत्व *adhimātratva* = शीघ्रः **rapid**

(vii) भवति *bhavati* = is, could be

(viii) ततः अपि *tataḥ api* = तेषु अधिकवेगः in these three, the rapid rate

(ix) विशेषः *viśeṣaḥ* = विशिष्यते excels

📖 **The speed of <u>concentration of mind</u> could be (i) slow, (ii) moderate or (iii) rapid, but in these three rates, the rapid rate excels.**

✍ Comments : The above mentioned rates of success in concentration of mind could be slow, moderate or rapid. The rapid success is best among the three rates.

1.23 ईश्वरप्रणिधानाद्वा ।

īśvaraprāṇidhānatvā *(īśvara-prāṇidhānat-vā)*

(i) वा *vā* = अथवा, अन्यथा or

(ii) ईश्वर-प्रणिधानात् *īśvara-prāṇidhānat* = ईश्वरं प्रति towards God

(iii) प्रणिधानात् *prāṇidhānat* = परित्यागात्, समर्पणात्, सर्वभावात् from full devotion

(iv) अपि *api* = also

(v) साधनाया: वेग: *sādhanāyāḥ vegaḥ* = the speed of concentration of mind

(vi) विशिष्यते *vishishyate* = excels.

📖 **Or, from full devotion towards God also the speed of concentration of mind excels.**

✍ Comments : One pointed devotion to God also speeds up the concentration of mind. This one pointed devotion is called the *ananya-yoga* (13:11) or *ananya-bhakti-yoga* (14:26) in the Gita.

अविपाक: ।

avipākaḥ

9. Non-desire in the fruit of *karma*

1.24 क्लेशकर्मविपाकाशयैरपरामृष्ट: पुरुषविशेष ईश्वर: ।

kleśakarmavipākāśayairaparāmarṣṭaḥ puruṣaviśeṣa īśvaraḥ

(kleśa-karma-vipākāśayair-aprāmarṣṭaḥ puruṣa-viśeṣa īśvaraḥfrom full devotion)

(o) क्लेश-कर्म-विपाक-आशयै: *kleśa-karma-vipākāśayaiḥ* =

(ii) क्लेशेन सह *kleśena saha* = अविद्यया सह च अस्मितया सह च रागेण सह च पीडया सह च द्वेषेण सह च अभिनिवेशेन च सह by perversion of mind, by insensitivity, by attachment, by affliction, by hatred and by fear of death, see 2.3

(ii) च *cha (and)*

(viii) कर्मणा सह *karmaṇaḥ saha* = पुण्येन सह च पापेन सह च पापपुण्याभ्यां सह च पापपुण्याभ्यां विना च by karma

(iv) च *cha* = and

(v) विपाकेन सह *vipākena saha* = कर्मफलेन वा कर्मफलवासनाया: सह by desire in the fruit of karma

(vi) च *cha* = and

(vii) इत्यादिनां समाहारेण सह *ityādinam samāhāreṇa saha* = with a combination of these three

(viii) अपरामृष्ट: *aparāmṛṣṭaḥ* = य: अबद्ध: अस्ति स: he who is unafflicted, indifferent, unattached, not coveting

(ix) पुरुषविशेष: *puruṣa viśeṣaḥ* = उत्तम: पुरुष: that supreme person

(x) 'ईश्वर:' *'īśvaraḥ'*

(xi) इति उच्यते *iti uchyate* = is known as, is called as

📖 **He who is not afflicted (i) by perversion of mind, (ii) by insensitivity, (iii) by attachment, (iv) by affliction, (v) by hatred, (vi) by fear of death; (vii) by *karma*, (viii) by desire in the fruit of *karma*, and (ix) by a combination of these, that supreme person is called *'īśvaraḥ.'***

✍ Comments : Ishvara is that supreme person, who is unaffected by affliction, hatred, fear of death, karma, and desire for fruit.

1.25 तत्र निरतिशयं सर्वज्ञबीजम् ।

tatra niratiśayam sarvajñabījam *(tatra nir-atiśatam sarvajña-bījam)*

(i) तत्र *tatra* = तं ईश्वरम् *tam Ishvaram* = to that supreme person

(o) सर्वज्ञ–बीजम् *sarvajña-bījam* =

(ii) तं सर्वज्ञं *tam sarvajñam* = यस्मिन् सर्वं ज्ञानं आप्यते परिसमाप्यते च तम् from whom in whom all knowledge originates and culminates

(iii) निरतिशयम् *nir-atiśayam* = न कश्चिदपि अतिशयं यस्मात् तम् whom nothing excels

(iv) 'निरतिशयं' *'niratiśayam'*

(v) आहुः *āhuḥ* = they call

📖 **(i) From whom and (ii) in whom all knowledge originates and culminates and (iii) than whom nothing excels, to that supreme person they call *'niratiśayam.'***

✍ Comments : That supreme person from whom all originates and in whom all dissolves, and who excels everything is *niratishaya*.

1.26 पूर्वेषामपि गुरुः कालेनानवच्छेदात् ।

pūrveṣāmapi guruḥ kālenānavachchhedāt

(pūrveṣām-api guruḥ kālenā-navachchhedāt)

(i) पूर्वेषाम् *pūrveṣām* = सः that supreme person

(ii) पूर्वजनानाम् *pūrvajānām* = than or of the predecessors

(iii) अपि *api* = also

(iv) गुरुः *guruḥ* = श्रेष्ठः, परमः, महान्, वरेण्यः, वरः, आर्यः is greater, superior

(v) यतः *yataḥ* = because

(vi) यस्य कालेन *yasya kālenān* = समयेन सह अपि for him with time also

(vii) अनवच्छेदात् *anavachchhedāt* = परिभाषाकरणात्, परिमिततायाः, मर्यादत्वात्, सीमिततायाः from the limitation

(viii) न भवितुम शक्यते *na anubhavitum shakyate* = is not possible, can not be there, is not there.

📖 **That supreme person is superior than the predecessors also, because for him limitation with time also is not there.**

✍ Comments : Being timeless not bound by time, that supreme person is superior to his predecessors also.

Being timeless, in Gita he is called *anādi* (10:3).

1.27 तस्य वाचकः प्रणवः ।

tasya vāćakaḥ praṇavaḥ *(tasya vāćakaḥ praṇavaḥ)*

(i) तस्य *tasya* = अतः तस्य ईश्वरस्य therefore for that supreme person

(ii) वाचकः *vāćakaḥ* = नाम, संज्ञा the title, mane

(iii) प्रणवः *praṇavaḥ* = 'ॐ,' ओम् 'Om'

(iv) इति ख्यातः *iti khyātaḥ* = is known as

📖 **Therefore, for that supreme person, the title is *'Om.'***

✍ Comments : Thus he is called Om. In Gita, this supreme person called *brahma* is the monosyllable "om" (8:13)

1.28 तज्जपस्तदर्थभावनम् ।

ta-jjapas-tadartha-bhāvanam *(tat-japaḥ-tadartha-bhāvanam)*

(i) तत् *tat* = तस्य ॐकारस्य of that 'Om' sound

(ii) जपः *japaḥ* = नामोच्चारणम् utterance

(iii) तद्-अर्थ-भावनम् *tadartha-bhāvanam* = तस्य अर्थः means, its meaning is

(iv) 'ईश्वरः' *Iśvaraḥ* = 'īśvaraḥ, saguṇa-brahma'

(v) इति अस्ति *iti asti* = is

(vi) इति चिन्तनीयम् *iti chintaniyam* = so one should think.

📖 **Utterance of that *'Om'* sound means *'īśvaraḥ,'* so one should think.**

✍ Comments : The sound of "Om" is Ishvara. This uttering of the Om is called *vyāharaṇam* in the Gita (8:13)

1.29 ततः प्रत्यक्चेतनाधिगमोऽप्यन्तरायाभावश्च ।

tataḥ pratyakćetanādhigamo'pyantarāyābhāvaśća

(tataḥ pratyak-ćetanā-dhigamo-'pya-ntarāyābhāvaḥ ća)

(i) ततः *tataḥ* = इति कृत्वा having done that utterance

(ii) अन्तराय *antarāya* = अन्तरायस्य, बाधायाः, विघ्नस्य of the obstacles

(iii) अभावः *abhāvaḥ* = अविद्यमानता disappearance

(iv) च *cha* = तथा as well as

(v) प्रत्यक्चेतनाधिगमः *pratyak-ćetanā-dhigaḥ* = अन्तरात्मनः स्वरूपस्य ज्ञानम् knowledge of self

(vi) अपि च भवति *api cha bhavati* = also occurs.

📖 **Having done that utterance, disappearance of obstacles as well as knowledge of self also occurs.**

✍ Comments : Utterance of "Om" causes (i) disappearance of obstacles and (ii) gives knowledge of self.

1.30 व्याधिस्त्यानसंशयप्रमादालस्याविरतिभ्रान्तिदर्शना-लब्धभूमिकत्वानवस्थितत्त्वानि चित्तविक्षेपास्तेन्तरायाः ।

vyādhistyānasam̐śayapramādālasyāviratibhrāntidarśanālabdhabhūmika tvānavasthitattvāni chittavikṣepāstentarāyāḥ

(vyādhi-styāna-sam̐śaya-pramād-ālasyāvirati-bhrānti-darśanālabdha-bhūmikatvānavasthi-t attvāni chitta-vikṣepās-te-antarāyāḥ)

(o) व्याधि–स्त्यान–संशय–प्रमाद–आलस्य–अविरति–भ्रान्ति–दर्शन–अलब्ध–भूमिकत्व–अनवस्थितत्त्वानि *vyādhi-styāna-sam̐śaya-pramād-ālasyā-virati-bhrānti-darśanā-labdha-bhūmikatva-anavasthitattvāni =*

(i) व्याधिः *vyādhiḥ* = रोगः, विपत्तिः, सङ्कटम् ailment

(ii) स्त्यानं *styānam* = अकर्मण्यता, निष्क्रियता inactivity

(iii) संशयः *samśayaḥ* = सन्देहः, विचिकित्सा, विकल्पः doubt, suspicion, skepticism

(iv) प्रमादः *pramādḥ* = अवलंबः, दीर्घसूत्रता, व्यापेक्षः procrastination

(v) आलस्यं *ālasyam* = तन्द्रिता, जाड्यम्, मान्द्यम् lethargy, laziness, idleness

(vi) अविरतिः *aviratiḥ* = आसक्तिः, अभिनिवेशः, अनुरागः attachment

(vii) भ्रन्ति-दर्शनं *bhrānti-darśanam* = मिथ्या-भावः, मूढ-ग्रहणम्, अपर्याय-बोधः, विसंवादः, असंमतिः delusion

(viii) अलब्ध-भूमिकत्वं *alabdha-bhūmikatvam* = असाफल्यम्, असिद्धिः, अपूर्णता, अकृतकार्यता failure

(ii) ते *te* = तानि = these, to these

(xiv) अन्तरायाः *antarāyāḥ* = विघ्नानि, बाधाः the obstacles

(xv) सन्ति *santi* = are.

📖 **Ailment, inactivity, skepticism, procrastination, lethargy, attachment, delusion, failure and wavering of mind, these are nine types of obstacles in loss of self-control.**

✍ Comments : With non-utterance of "Om," the resulting loss of self control causes : (i) Ailment, (ii) inactivity, (iii) skepticism, (iv) procrastination, (v) lethargy, (vi) attachment, (vii) delusion, (viii) failure, and (ix) wavering of mind, (and) ...

1.31 दुःखदौर्मनस्याङ्गमेजयत्वश्वासप्रश्वासा विक्षेपसहभुवः ।

duḥkhadaurmanasyāṅgamejayatva-śvāsa-praśvāsā vikśepasahabhuvaḥ

(duḥkha-daurmanasyā-ṅgamejayatva-śvāsa-praśvāsā vikśepa-saha-bhuvaḥ)

(o) दुःख-दौर्मनस्य-अङ्गमेजयत्व-श्वास-प्रश्वासाः *duḥkha-daurmanasya-aṅgamejayatva-śvāsa-praśvāsāḥ* =

(i) दुःखं *duḥkham* = क्लेशः, बाधा, व्यथा, क्रच्छ्रम्, तापः sorrow, pain

(ii) दौर्मनस्यं *daurmanasyam* = मनसः क्षोभः, मनःसन्तापः anguish

(viii) अङ्गमेजयत्वं *aṅgamejayatvam* = अङ्गेषु विकम्पनम् jitter, cramp

(iv) श्वास-प्रश्वासौ *śvāsa- praśvāsau* = निर्बन्धितं श्वासोच्छ्वसनं च unregulated breathing

(v) विक्षेप-सह-भुवः *vikśepa-saha-bhuvaḥ* = विक्षेपेण सह, संयमस्य अभावेन, चित्तस्य निपातेन with the lack of self control

(vi) भवन्ति च *bhavanti cha* = also occur.

📖 **With the lack of self-control also occur sorrow, anguish, jitter and unregulated breathing.**

✍ Comments : (continued from the previous) ...and (x) sorrow, (xi) anguish, (xii) jitter, and (xiii) unregulated breathing.

1.32 तत्प्रतिषेधार्थमेकतत्त्वाभ्यासः ।

tat-pratiṣedhārtham-eka-tattvābhyāsaḥ

(tat-pratiṣedhārtham-eka-tattvābhyāsaḥ)

(i) तत् *tat* = तान् विक्षेपान् those obstacles

(ii) प्रतिषेधार्थम् *pratiṣedhārtham* = निवारणाय, अवरोधार्थम् for warding off, expulsion

(iii) एक-तत्त्व *eka-tattva* = एकाग्रतया, एकचित्तेन, एकचेतसा with one-pointed, undiverted mind

(iv) अभ्यासः *abhyāsaḥ* = practice

(v) आवश्यकः *āvashyakaḥ* = is required.

📖 **For warding off those obstacles, practice with one-pointed mind is required.**

✍ Comments : for removing these 13 obstacles, one-pointed devotion is required. In Gita it is called *ekāgram* (6:12).

1.33 मैत्रीकरुणामुदितोपेक्षाणां सुखदुःखपुण्यापुण्यविषयाणां भावनातश्चित्तप्रसादनम् ।

maitrīkaruṇāmuditopekṣaṇām sukhadu:khapuṇyāpuṇyaviṣayāṇām bhāvanātaścittaprasādanam

maitrī-karuṇāmudito-pekṣaṇām sukha-du:kha-puṇyāpuṇya-viṣayāṇām bhāvanāta-ścitta-prasādanam)

(o) सुख-दुःख-पुण्य-अपुण्य-विषयाणाम् *sukha-du:kha-puṇya-apuṇya-viṣayāṇām* =

(i) सुखं *sukham* = निवृत्तिः, शान्तिः, सन्तोषः happiness

(ii) दुःखं *du:kham* = क्लेशः, तापः unhappiness

(iii) पुण्यम् *puṇyam* = सुकृतम्, भद्रम्, मङ्गलम् righteous consequence

(iv) अपुण्यं *apuṇya* = पापम्, दुष्कृतम्, किल्बिषम्, वृजिनम्, कल्मषम्, एनः, दुरितम्, शल्यम् unrighteous consequence

(v) इत्यादिकानां *ityādinām* = etc.

(vi) विषयाणाम् *vishayāṇām* = व्यापाराणाम् of such concerns

(o) मैत्री-करुणा-मुदिता-उपेक्षाणाम् *maitrī-karuṇā-muditā-pekṣaṇām* =

(vi) मैत्री *maitrī* = मित्रता, सख्यम्, सौहार्दम् friendship, amity

(vii) करुणा *karuṇā* = कृपा, दया, अनुकम्पा compassion

(viii) मुदिता *muditā* = प्रसन्नता, उल्लासः, तोषः, आह्लादः joy

(ix) उपेक्षा *upekṣā* = औदासिन्यम्, निःस्पएहता, तटस्थता, निःसङ्गता sorrow

(x) इत्यादिकानाम् *ityādinām* = of shch as

(xi) भावनातः *bhāvanātaḥ* = भावनावशात्, चिन्तनेन, विमर्शेन, विचारेण with the contemplation

(xi) चित्त-प्रसादनम् *citta-prasādanam* = चेतसः शुद्धिः निर्मलता, विमलता, पवित्रता purity of mind

(xii) भवति *bhavati* = occurs.

📖 **Purity of mind occurs with the contemplation of such concerns as happiness, unhappiness, righteous consequence, unrighteous consequence, amity, compassion, joy, sorrow ...etc.**

✍ Comments : Contemplation of such concerns as : (i) happiness, (ii) unhappiness, (iii) righteous consequence, (iv) unrighteous consequence, (v) amity, (vi) compassion, (vii) joy, (viii) sorrow, etc. causes purity of mind. In Gita (13:8) such concern is an aspect of knowledge.

1.34 प्रच्छर्दनविधारणाभ्यां वा प्राणस्य ।

prac̍hhardanavidhāraṇābhyām vā prāṇasya

(prac̍hhardana-vidhāraṇābhyām vā prāṇasya)

(i) वा *vā* = च and

(ii) प्राणस्य *prāṇasya* = श्वास-उच्छ्वासस्य of breath

(iii) प्रच्छर्दन-विधारणाभ्याम् *prac̍hhardana-vidhāraṇābhyām* = प्रच्छर्दनेन, नि:श्वसनेन by exhalation

(iv) च *cha* = and

(v) विधारणेन *vidhāraṇena* = उच्छ्वसनेन च by exhalation also

(vi) चित्त-प्रसादनम् *c̍itta-prasādanam* = चेतस: प्रसादनं, शुद्धि:, पावित्र्यं purification of mind

(vii) भवति *bhavati* = occurs

📖 **And, by inhalation and exhalation of breath also purification of mind occurs.**

✍ Comments : Purification of mind also with regulated inhalation and exhalation of breath.

1.35 विषयवती वा प्रवृत्तिरुत्पन्ना मनस: स्थितिनिबन्धनी ।

viṣayavatī vā pravṛttirutpannā manasaḥ sthitinibandhanī

(viṣayavatī vā pravṛtti-rutpannā manasaḥ sthiti-nibandhanī)

(i) विषयवती *viṣayavatī* = उपरोक्तानां विषयेषु , उपरोक्तानां व्यापारेषु in above mentioned concerns;

योगिन: *yoginaḥ* = of yogī;

प्रवृत्ति: *pravṛttiḥ* = शीलता inclination, liking of the yogi

(ii) उत्पन्ना *utpannā* = उत्पन्ना भूत्वा *utpannā bhūtvā* = arose, having grown

(iii) वा *vā* = अथवा सा शीलता and that inclination

(iv) मनस: *manasaḥ* = चित्तस्य of mind

(v) स्थिति: *sthiti* = अवस्था **the state**

(vi) निबन्धनी *nibandhanī* = संयमिनी **steady**

(vii) भवति *bhavati* = becomes.

📖 **And, inclination of *yogī* having grown in above mentioned concerns, the state of mind becomes steady.**

✍ Comments : The concerns mentioned in the above two sutras, cause steady state of mind. In Gita it is called *sthitā-dhī* or *sthitadhī* (2:54)

1.36 विशोका वा ज्योतिष्मती ।

viśokā vā jyotiṣmati *(viśokā vā jyotiṣ-mati)*

(i) वि-शोका *viśokā* = सा विशोका, शोक-रहिता that sorrowless state, that steady state

(ii) योगिन: *jyoginaḥ* = of the yogi

(iii) ज्योतिष्मती *jyotiṣ-mati* = प्रकाशमया प्रवृति: enlightened state

(iv) वा *jyotiṣ-mati-vā* = अपि also

(v) भवति *bhavati* = becomes

📖 **And, with that steady state, the *yogī* becomes enlightened one.**

✍ Comments : The yogi with steady state of mind is an enlightened yogi. In Gita he is called *sthitadhīḥ* (2:56)

1.37 वीतरागविषयं वा चित्तम् ।

vītarāgaviṣayam vā ćittam *(vīta-rāga-viṣayam vā ćittam)*

(i) वा *vā* = च = and thus

(ii) चित्तम् *ćittam* = मनः, चेतः mind, mind of the yogī

(o) वीतरागविषयम् *vīta-rāga-viṣayam* =

(iii) वीतं *vītam* = निवृत्तं, गतं, विगतं departed

(iv) राग *rāga* = अनुरक्तिः, अनुरागः, आसक्तिः attachment

(v) विषयात् *viṣayāt* = व्यापारात् from those concerns

(vi) भवति *bhavati* = becomes

And, thus mind of the *yogī* becomes departed from attachment to those concerns.

Comments : And then such yogi of enlightened mind becomes detached from attachment. Such detached yogi is called *muni* in the Gita (2:56).

1.38 स्वप्ननिद्राज्ञानालम्बनं वा ।

svapnanidrājñānālambanam vā *(svapna-nidrā-jñānā-lambanam vā)*

(o) स्वप्न-निद्रा-ज्ञान-अलम्बनम् *svapna-nidrā-jñānā-lambanam* =

(i) तस्य योगिनः *tasya yoginaḥ* = of the yogī

(ii) स्वप्नं *svapna* = आभासः, प्रसुप्त-ज्ञानम् intuition, gut feeling, instinct, sixth sense

(iii) निद्रा *nidrā* = स्वपनम्, सुप्तिः, स्वापः slumber, siesta

(iv) ज्ञान *jñānā* = भावः, प्रतीतिः, बोधः awareness, perception, discrement, grasp, understanding

(v) अलम्बनं *alambanam* = विश्वासः, ग्रहणम्, धारणम् conviction, belief

(vi) वा *vā* = and

(vii) चित्तं *chittam* = mind

(viii) स्थिरं *sthiram* = stable, unwavering, established

(ix) करोति *karoti* = it makes

And, it makes the (i) sixth sense, (ii) siesta, (iii) perception, (iv) conviction,

(v) belief and (vi) the mind of the *yogī* unwavering.

✍ Comments : The steady state of mind makes the mind of the yogi unwavering. Such unwavering yogi is called *sthitaprajña* in the Gita (2:55).

1.39 यथाभिमतध्यानाद्वा ।

yathābhimatadhyānādvā *(yathā-bhimata-dhyānād-vā)*

(i) वा *vā* = च and

(o) यथा–अभिमत–ध्यानात् *yathā-bhimata-dhyānāt* =

(ii) यथा *yathā* = यावत् which, as

(iii) अभिमत *abhimata* = अनुकूलम्, हितकरम् optimum, most suitable

(iv) भवेत् *bhavet* = may be

(v) तावत् *tāvat* = that, so

(vi) ध्यानात् *dhyānāt* = समाधिना by meditating on, by focusing on

(vii) चित्तं *chittam* = mind

(viii) स्थिरं *sthiram* = stable, unwavering, established

(ix) भवति *bhavati* = becomes.

🕮 **And, by meditating on that which may be most suitable, mind becomes unwavering.**

✍ Comments : Mind also becomes unwavering by meditating on the most suitable object.

1.40 परमाणुपरममहत्त्वान्तोऽस्य वशीकारः ।

paramāṇuparamamahattvānto'sya vaśīkaraḥ

(paramāṇu-parama-mahattvānto'sya vaśī-karaḥ)

(i) अस्य *asya* = of this, of this meditation

(o) परमाणु–परम–महत्त्वान्तः *paramāṇu-parama-mahattvāntaḥ* =

(ii) परमाणुतः *paramāṇutaḥ* = सूक्ष्मांशतः, लघुत्तमाङ्गतः from even a small amount, degree

(iii) परम–महत्त्वान्तः *parama-mahattvāntaḥ* = महत्तमाङ्ग–पर्यन्तम् to large amount, degree

(iv) अपि *api* = also

(v) वशीकरः *vaśīkaraḥ* = वशीकारी conducive to

(vi) मनोनिग्रहकारी *manonigrahakarī* = self-control

(vii) भवति *bhavati* = becomes

📖 **Also, from even a small degree to a large degree of this meditation, becomes conducive to self-control.**

✍ Comments : Meditation is conducive to self control. Meditation is called *dhyānam* in the Gita (12:12)

समापत्तिः ।

samāpattiḥ

10. Oneness

1.41 क्षीणवृत्तेरभिजातस्येव मणेर्ग्रहितृग्रहणग्राह्येषु तत्स्थतदञ्जनता समापत्तिः ।

kṣīṇavṛtterabhijātasyeva maṇergrahitṛgrahaṇagrāhyeṣu tatsthatadañjanatā samāpattiḥ

(kṣīṇa-vṛtter-abhijātasy-eva maṇer-grahitṛ-grahaṇa-grāhyeṣu tat-stha-tad-añjanatā samāpattiḥ)

(i) क्षीणवृत्तेः *kṣīṇa-vṛtteḥ* =

(ii) यस्य *yasya* = he whose

(iii) वृत्तिः *vṛttiḥ* = चित्तावस्था = state of mind

(iv) क्षीणा *kṣīṇa* = अविचला, शान्ता, स्थिरा serene, tranquil, quiet

(v) जाता *jātā* = has become

(vi) तस्य *tasya* = his

(vii) मणेः-इव *maṇeḥ iva* = स्फटिकवत् like a clear crystal

(viii) अभिजातस्य *abhijātasy* = निर्मलं जातस्य untainted, purified

(ix) चित्तस्य *chittasy* = mind

(o) ग्रहितृ-ग्रहण-ग्राह्येषु *grahitṛ-grahaṇa-grāhyeṣu* =

(x) ग्रहितृ *grahitṛ* = ग्रहिता पुरुषः receptor purusha

(xi) ग्रहण *grahaṇa* = मनादीनि इन्द्रियाणि six organs of reception including mind

(xii) ग्राह्य *grāhya* = पञ्च-भूतानि च विषयाः च and five primary elements and their objects to be recepted

(xiii) आदिषु *ādishu* = in ...etc.

(o) तत्स्थ-तद्-अञ्जनता *tat-stha-tad-añjanatā* =

(xiv) तत्र स्थितं चित्तं *tatra sthitam chittam* = the mind that came in contact with

(xv) स्थिरं *sthiram* = stable

(xvi) च *cha* = and

(xvii) तदाकारं च *tadākāram* = तद्रूपम्, तत्समम् and of same attributes, of oneness

(xviii) भवति *bhavati* = becomes

📖 **He whose state of mind has become tranquil, his untainted mind, that came in contact with (i) receptor *puruṣa,* (ii) six organs of reception and the (iii) five primary elements (iv) and their objects to be receipted, becomes stable and 'one' with those contacts, like a clear crystal.**

✍ Comments : The tranquil and untainted state of crystal clear mind becomes one with *purusha*. In Gita such yogi is called *brahmabhūta* (5:24).

1.42 तत्र शब्दार्थज्ञानविकल्पैः सङ्कीर्णा सवितर्का समापत्तिः ।

tatra śabdārthajñānavikalpaiḥ saṅkīrṇā savitarkā samāpattiḥ

(tatra śabdārtha-jñāna-vikalpaiḥ saṅkīrṇā sa-vitarkā samāpattiḥ)

(i) तत्र *tatra* = तस्मिन् in that state

(o) शब्दार्थ–ज्ञान–विकल्पैः *śabdārtha-jñāna-vikalpaiḥ* =

(ii) शब्द *śabda* = शब्दादि–विषयैः senses such as hearing, sight etc.

(iii) अर्थ *artha* = अर्थादि–विषयैः objects such as purpose

(iv) ज्ञान *jñāna* = ज्ञानादि–विकल्पै contrivances as perception or conviction

(v) च *cha* = and

(vi) सङ्कीर्णा *saṅkīrṇā* = युक्ता equipped with

(vii) समापत्तिः *samāpattiḥ* = एकता, तदाकारता oneness

(viii) 'सवितर्का' *sa-vitarkā* = 'savitarkā' samādhi, tainted samādhi

(ix) इति उच्यते *iti uchyate* = is known as, is called as

📖 **That state of mind, which has oneness with (i) senses such as hearing, (ii) objects such as purpose, and (iii) contrivances such as perception, is known as *'savitarkā' (tainted) samādhi.***

✍ Comments : Such meditation equipped with senses, objects and perceptions is called *sa-vitarka samadhi.*

1.43 स्मृतिपरिशुद्धौ स्वरूपशून्येवार्थमात्रनिर्भासा निर्वितर्का ।

smṛtipariśuddhau svarūpaśūnyevārthamātranirbhāsā nirvitarkā

(smṛti-pari-śuddhau svarūpa-śūnye-vārtha-mātra-nirbhāsā nir-vitarkā)

(i) स्मृति–परिशुद्धौ *smṛti-pari-śuddhau* = शब्दादि विषयैः the aspects such as hearing, sight etc.

(ii) च प्रतीत्या *cha pratītyā* = and conviction

(iii) च विरहिता *cha virahitā* = not in, without

(iv) शुद्धा *śuddhā* = the pure

(v) स्मृतौ *smritau* = in the reminiscence, recollection, remembrance

(o) स्वरूप-शून्या *svarūpa-śūnyā* =

(vi) स्वरूप *svarūpa* = मूल-रूपेण *muīla-rūpeṇa* with the original form

(vii) शून्या *śūnyā* = विरहिता, रिक्ता = devoid

(viii) इव *iva* = सदृशी = such

(ix) अर्थमात्र-निर्भासा *artha-mātra-nirbhāsā* = वितर्कहीना, निर्मोहा, नि:संदेहा doubtless, one pointed

(x) चित्तावस्था *chittāvasthā* = state of mind

(xi) निर्-र्वितर्का *nirvitarkā* = 'निर्वितर्का समाधि:' 'nirvitarkā samādhi' or untainted samādhi

(xii) इति उच्यते *iti uchyate* = is known as, is called as

📖 **When the aspects such as hearing and conviction are not in the reminiscence, such emptied, pure in the original form and one pointed state of mind is called as *'nirvitarkā (untainted) samādhi'***

✍ Comments : The meditation, with the mind in one pointed original state, is called *nir-vitarka* samadhi. Such meditation is called *ekāgram* in the Gita (6:12-13).

1.44 एतयैव सविचारा निर्विचारा च सूक्ष्मविषया व्याख्याता ।

etayaiva savićārā nirvićārā ća sūkṣmaviṣayā vyākhyātā

(etayā-eva sa-vićārā nir-vićārā ća sūkṣma-viṣayā vyākhyātā)

(i) एतया एव *etayā-eva* = सवितर्का वा निर्वितर्का इति संज्ञया with the names as 'savitarkā' and 'nirvitarkā'

(ii) पूर्वोक्ता *pūrvoktā* = previously described

(iii) समाधि: *samādhiḥ* = the samādhi

(iv) सूक्ष्म-विषया *sūkṣma-viṣayā* = सूक्ष्म-विषयसम्बन्धिनी relating to the subtle aspects

(v) सविचारा *sa-vićārā* = विचारपूर्वका samādhi with discrimination

(vi) निर्विचारा च *nir-vićārā cha* = विचारहीना samādhi without discrimination

(vii) इति व्याख्याते *iti vikhyāte* = वर्णिते known as

(viii) स्तः *sthạ* = are

📖 **The <u>*samādhi*</u> previously described with the names as *'savitarkā'* and *'nirvitarkā'* relating to the subtle aspects, are also known as *'savichārā,'* i.e. *samādhi* with discrimination and *'nirvichārā,'* i.e. *samādhi* without discrimination.**

1.45 सूक्ष्मविषयत्वं चालिङ्गपर्यवसानम् ।

sūkṣmaviṣayatvam ćāliṅgaparyavasānam

(sūkṣma-viṣayatvam ćāliṅga-paryavasānam)

(i) च *ća* = And

(ii) सूक्ष्म-विषयत्वम् *sūkṣma-viṣayatvam* = subtle subject

(iii) प्रकृतेः *prakṛteḥ* = of the 'pṛkṛti,' of 'the five primary elements and three attributes'

(iv) सूक्ष्मत्वं *sūkṣmatvam* = गूढत्वम् the ubtleness

(v) अलिङ्ग-पर्यवसानम् *aliṅga-paryavasānam* = दृष्ट-द्रव्येषु in the visible aspects

(vi) सूक्ष्मतमम् *sūkṣmatamam* = subtle

(vii) अस्ति *asti* = is

(viii) खलु *khalu* = indeed

📖 **And, the subtleness of 'the <u>five primary elements and the three attributes</u>' in the visible aspects is indeed subtle.**

✍ Comments : The five *bhutas* and the three *gunas* are subtle in the visible beings.

1.46 ता एव सबीजः समाधिः ।

tā eva sabījaḥ samādhiḥ *(tāḥ eva sa-bīja samādhiḥ)*

(i) ताः एव *tā eva* = ताः सर्वाः these all

(ii) समाधयः *samadhayaḥ* = *samādhis* see 1.41-45

(iii) समाहारेण *samāhāreṇa* = collectively, the group of

(iv) 'सबीज-समाधिः' *'sabīja-samādhi'* = samadhi with safeguard

(v) बीज bīja = आश्रयः shelter, safeguard

(vi) इति उच्यते *iti uchyate* = is known as, is called as

📖 **The group of all these *samādhis* is collectively called as *'sabīja-samādhi'***

✍ Comments : The above mentioned four samadhis (*sa-vitarka, nir-vitarka, sa-vichara, nir-vichara*) are collectively called *sa-beej-samaadhi* i.e. Samadhi with a safeguard.

1.47 निर्विचारवैशारद्येऽध्यात्मप्रसादः ।

nirvićāravaiśāradye'dhyātmaprasādaḥ

(nir-vićāra-vaiśāradye-'dhyātma-prasādaḥ)

(i) निर्विचार-वैशारद्ये *nir-vićāra-vaiśāradye* = निर्विचार-समाधिः the 'nirvichāra-samādhi' the samādhi without discrimination see 1.44↑

(ii) निर्मलत्वात् *nirmalatvāt* = because of its purity

(iii) अध्यात्म-प्रसादः *adhyātma-prasādaḥ* = अध्यात्मप्रसादं, ब्रह्मज्ञानस्य आनन्दम्, आत्मज्ञानस्य समाधानम् the joy of self realization

(iv) ददाति *dadāti* = gives

📖 **The *samādhi* without discrimination, because of its purity, gives the joy of Self Realization.**

✍ Comments : The purity of nir-vichara *samadhi* gives joy of self realization.

1.48 ऋतम्भरा तत्र प्रज्ञा ।

ṛtambharā tatra prajñā (*ṛtambharā tatra prajñā*)

(i) तत्र *tatra* = तस्याः समाधौ in that samadhi

(ii) प्रज्ञा *prajñā* = बुद्धिः, योगिनः मतिः the mind of the yogī, the thinking of the yogī

(iii) 'ऋतम्भरा' *ṛtambharā'* = सत्य धारिणी, यथार्थ धारिणी चित्तवृत्तिः 'ṛtambharā' i.e. meaningful

(iv) ऋतम् *ṛtam* = यथार्थ truth, true meaning;

(v) भरा *bharā* = धारिणी bearer

(vi) इति उच्यते *iti uchyate* = is known as, is called as

📖 **In that *samādhi*, the thinking of the *yogī* is *ṛtambharā'* i.e. meaningful.**

✍ Comments : The *nir-vichara samadhi* is of meaningful thinking.

1.49 श्रुतानुमानप्रज्ञाभ्यामन्यविषया विशेषार्थात् ।

śrutānumānaprajñābhyāmanyaviṣayā viśeṣārthāt

(śrutānumāna-prajñābhyām-anya-viṣayā viśeṣā-rthāt)

(o) श्रुत–अनुमान–प्रज्ञाभ्याम् *śrutānumāna-prajñābhyām* =

(i) श्रुतायाः *śrutāyāḥ* = आकर्णितायाः, श्रवणगोचरिकृतायाः than the thought arose as a result of what is heard

(ii) च अनुमानितायाः *cha anumānitāyāḥ* = तर्कसाधितायाः and the thought as a result of logic

(iii) च अपेक्षया *cha apekshyāḥ* = than

(iv) प्राज्ञाभ्याम् *prajñābhyām* = बुद्धिभ्याम्, मतिभ्याम्, मनसोः than the other two thoughts

(v) अन्यविषया *anya-viṣayā* = यस्याः बुद्धेः विषयाः भिन्नाः the aspects of such ṛtambharā thinking are different than

(o) विशेषार्थात् *viśeṣā-rthāt* =

(vi) येन *yena* = because, by which

(vii) एषा *eshā* = this ṛtambharā thinking, the meaningful thinking

(viii) विशेष–अर्थयुक्ता *vishesha-arthayuktā* = equipped with more definite purpose

(ix) अस्ति *asti* = is

The aspects of such (i) *ṛtambharā* thinking are different than (ii) the thought arose as a result of what is heard and (iii) the thought as a result of logic. Because, this *ṛtambharā* thinking is equipped with more definite purpose than the other two thoughts.

Comments : *Ritambhara* thinking, being meaningful reasoning, is superior to that based on what is heard and what the logic says.

1.50 तज्जः संस्कारोऽन्यसंस्कारप्रतिबन्धी ।

tajjaḥ saṁskāro'anyasaṁskārapratibandhī

(taj-jaḥ saṁskāro-'anya-saṁskāra-pratibandhī)

(i) तत्–जः *taj-jaḥ* = यः संस्कारः तस्मात् प्रज्ञायाः जायते the impression on mind that that is borne as a result of the ṛtambharā thinking

(ii) संस्कारः *saṁskāraḥ* = सः संस्कारः, मानसी शिक्षा, शिक्षा–प्रभावः that impression on mind

(o) अन्य–संस्कार–प्रतिबन्धी *anya-saṁskāra-pratibandhī* =

(iii) अन्येषां *anya-saṁ* = of other influences

(iv) संस्काराणां *saṁskārāṇām* = influences, impressions

(v) प्रतिबन्धकारकः *pratibandhakārakaḥ* = prohibitor

(vi) भवति *bhavati* = becomes

The impression on mind that that is borne as a result of the *ṛtambharā*

(meaningful) thinking, that influence on mind becomes the prohibitor of other influences.

✍ Comments : And therefore, the rithambhara thinking prohibits other influences on mind. Ritambhara thinking is the meaningful thinking.

1.51 तस्यापि निरोधे सर्वनिरोधान्निर्बिजः समाधिः ।

tasyāpi nirodhe sarvanirodhānnirbījaḥ samādhiḥ

(tasyā-pi nirodhe sarva-nirodhān-nir-bījaḥ samādhiḥ)

(i) तस्य *tasya* = तस्य अन्यसंस्कारस्य, ऋतम्भरा चित्तवृत्तेः संस्कारस्य of the impression of the ṛtambharā thinking

(ii) निरोधे *nirodhe* = प्रतिबन्धः भूत्वा on prohibiting

(iii) अपि *api* = अपि च also

(iv) सर्व-निरोधात् *sarva-nirodhāt* = सर्वेभ्यः संस्कारेभ्यः प्रतिबन्धात् as a result of prohibition of all influences

(v) निर्बिजः *nir-bījaḥ* = निर्बिज-संस्कारस्य without any seed or without any source of influence

(vi) सा *sā* = that samādhi

(vii) समाधिः *samādhiḥ* = 'निर्बिज-समाधिः' 'nirbīja-samādhi'

(viii) इति उच्यते *iti uchyate* = is known as, is called as

📖 **On prohibiting the impression of the *ṛtambharā* thinking also, as a result of prohibition of all influences, that <u>*samādhi* without any source of influence</u>, is called as *'nirbīja-samādhi.'***

✍ Comments : If the meditation is done without *ritambhara* (meaningful) thinking, that meditation is called *nir-beeja-samadhi.* The *beeja* means a source.

2. साधनापादः ।

Sādhanāpādaḥ

क्रियायोगः ।

11. Discipline of right actions

2.1 तपः स्वाध्यायेश्वरप्रणिधानानि क्रियायोगः ।

tapaḥ svādhyāyeśvarapraṇidhāni kriyāyogaḥ

(tapaḥ svādhyāye-śvara-praṇidhāni kriyā-yogaḥ)

(o) तप–स्वाध्याय–ईश्वर–प्रणिधानानि *tapaḥ svādhyāye-śvara-praṇidhāni* =

(i) तपः = स्वधर्मस्य स्वगुणानुसारेण सर्वदा पालनम् austerity of performing righteous actions according to one's own inborn nature

(ii) स्वाध्यायः *svādhyaḥ* = शास्त्राभ्यासः study of scriptures

(iii) ईश्वर–प्रणिधानं *iśvara-praṇidhānam* = ईश्वरं प्रति श्रद्धा, निष्ठा, भक्तिः devotion to God

(iv) च *cha* = and

(v) 'क्रियायोगः' *kriyā-yoga* = the discipline of right actions, 'kriyā-yoga'

(vi) इति उच्यते *iti uchyate* = is known as, is called as

📖 **The discipline of austerity of performing righteous actions according to (i) one's own inborn nature, (ii) study of scriptures and (iii) devotion to God, is called as *'kriyā-yoga.'***

✍ Comments : The yoga of performing righteous actions according to ones own inborn nature and devotion is *kriya-yoga.* In Gita (18.47) it is called *svabhava-niyatam karma* or *karma-yoga.*

2.2 समाधिभावनार्थः क्लेशतनूकरणार्थश्च ।

samādhibhavanārthaḥ kleśatanūkaraṇārthaśca

(samādhi-bhavanārthaḥ kleśa-tanū-karaṇārthaḥ ća)

i) क्लेश-तनू-करणार्थः *kleśa-tanū-karaṇārthaḥ* = एषः उपरोक्तः क्रियायोगः this above mentioned kriyāyoga

ii) क्लेषानां *kleśānām* = of sorrow, grief, pains, afflictions

iii) क्षिणकारकः *kṣiṇakārakaḥ* = attenuator

iv) च *cha* = as well as

(o) समाधि-भावनार्थः *samādhi-bhavanārthaḥ* =

(v) समाधेः *samādheḥ* = for the samādhi

(vi) भावनार्थः *bhavanārthaḥ* = state of mind

(vii) सिद्धिकारः *siddhikārahh* = giver of success

(viii) अस्ति *asti* = is

📖 **This above mentioned *kriyā-yoga* is attenuator of afflictions as well as giver of state of mind for success for the *samādhi.***

✍ Comments : The *kriya-yoga* (karma-yoga) is conducive to the success of yoga.

क्लेशः ।

kleśaḥ

12. Affliction

2.3 अविद्यास्मितारागद्वेषाभिनिवेशाः क्लेशाः ।

avidyāsmitārāgadveṣābhiniveśāḥ kleśāḥ

(a-vidyāsmitārāga-dveṣābhiniveśāḥ kleśāḥ)

(o) अविद्या-अस्मिता-राग-द्वेष-अभिनिवेशाः *a-vidyāsmitārāga-dveṣābhiniveśāḥ* =

(i) अविद्या *a-vidyā* = अज्ञानम्, जाड्यम् perversion of mind

(ii) अस्मिता *asmitā* = अभेदः illusion of indifference

(iii) रागः *rāgaḥ* = अनुरागः, अनुरक्तिः, आसक्तिः, प्रीतिः attachment

(iv) द्वेषः *dveṣaḥ* = नानुरागः, अप्रीतिः, द्वंद्वभावः hatred, dislike

(v) च *cha* = and

(vi) अभिनिवेशः *abhiniveśāḥ* = जीवनस्य तीव्रा वासना, मृत्योः भयात् क्लेशः ardent longing for being alive, fear of death

(vii) इति पञ्च *iti pancha* = five

(viii) 'क्लेशाः' *kleśāḥ* = afflictions

(ix) सन्ति *santi* = are

📖 **(i) Perversion of mind, (ii) illusion of indifference, (iii) attachment, (iv) hatred and (v) ardent longing for being alive are five *'kleṣās'* (afflictions).**

✍ Comments : *Klesha* is the group of five afflictions. The afflictions are : (i) perversion of mind, (ii) illusion of indifference, (iii) attachment, (iv) hatred (v) longing to be alive.

अविद्या ।

avidyā

13. The Influenced State of Mind

2.4 अविद्या क्षेत्रमुत्तरेषां प्रसुप्ततनुविच्छिन्नोदाराणाम् ।

avidyā kṣetram-uttareṣām prasupta-tanu-vićhhinno-dārāṇām

(avidyā kṣetram-uttareṣām prasupta-tanu-vićhhinno-dārāṇām)

(o) प्रसुप्त-तनु-विच्छिन्न-उदाराणाम् *prasupta-tanu-vićhhinno-dārāṇām* =

(i) प्रसुप्तस्य *prasuptasya* = सुप्यस्य, छन्नस्य, अप्रकाशस्य, अन्तर्हितस्य, निभृतस्य of latent

i) तनोः *tanoḥ* = क्षीणस्य, निरुद्यमस्य, अव्यवसायस्य, निष्क्रियस्य तनोः of inactive body

ii) विच्छिन्नस्य *vićhhinnsya* = निगृहितस्य, रुद्धस्य, निगूढस्य, स्तम्भितस्य, समुपोढस्य of suppressed

v) उदाराणां *udārāṇām* = अतिरिक्तस्य, प्रबलस्य, प्रधानस्य of dominant nature

v) च *cha* = and

vi) इति चतस्त्राणाम् *iti chatasrāṇam* = of these four kinds

vii) उत्तरेषाम् *uparesham* = उपरोक्तायाः अस्मितायाः रागस्य च द्वेषस्य च अभिनिवेशस्य च for the previously mentioned four afflictions namely indifference, attachment, hatred and fear of death see 1.24↑

viii) क्षेत्रम् *kṣetram* = कारणम् the cause

ix) 'अविद्या' = 'avidyā,' the influenced state of mind, The Influenced State of Mind

x) एव अस्ति *eva asti* = is only

📖 **The cause for the previously mentioned four afflictions (namely : insensitivity, attachment, hatred and fear of death) that are of four kinds (namely : latent, inactive, suppressed or dominant) is *'avidyā'* (the influenced state of mind) only.**

✍ Comments : *Avidya* is influenced state of mind. It is the cause for afflictions.

2.5 अनित्याशुचिदुःखानात्मसु नित्यशुचिसुखात्मख्यातिरविद्या ।

anityāśuchiduḥkhānātmasu nityaśuciśukhātmakhyātiravidyā

(anityāśuchi-duḥkhānātmasu nitya-śući-sukhātma-khyātir-avidyā)

(o) अनित्य-अशुचि-दुःख-अनात्मसु *anityāśuchi-duḥkhānātmasu* =

(i) अनित्यम् *anityam* = अस्थायि, असत्यम् impermanent

(ii) अशुचिः *aśuchi* = अपवित्रम्, अधार्मिकं, अशुच्यम् unrighteous

(iii) दुःखं *duḥkham* = तापः, क्लेशः suffering

(iv) अनात्म *anātma* = शारीरिकं, देहिकं manifest

(v) आदिषु *ādishu* = in ...etc.

(o) नित्य-शुचि-सुख-आत्म-ख्याति *nitya-śucí-sukhātma-khyāti* =

(vi) नित्यं *nityam* = स्थायि, सत्यम् permanence

(vii) शुचिः *śuchiḥ* = पवित्रम्, धार्मिकं, शुद्धम् righteousness

(viii) सुखं *sukham* = निवृत्तिः, शान्तिः happiness

(ix) आत्म *ātma* = आत्मतत्त्वं the unmanifest

(x) ख्यातिः *khyātiḥ* = अनुभूतिः the perception

(xi) 'अविद्या' *'avidya'* = perversion of mind, ihe Influenced State of Mind

(xii) इति उच्यते *iti uchyate* = is known as, is called as

(i) The perception of permanence in impermanent, (ii) righteousness in unrighteous, (iii) happiness in suffering and (iv) manifest in the un-manifest ...etc., is called as *'avidyā* (perversion of mind).'

Comments : A negative of false perception is *Avidya*.

अस्मिता ।

asmitā

14. Delusion of Indifference

2.6 दृग्दर्शनशक्त्योरेकात्मतेवास्मिता ।

dṛgdarśanaśaktyo'rekātmatevāsmitā

(dṛg-darśana-śaktyo-'rekātmatevā-smitā)

(o) दृक्-दर्शन-शक्त्योः *dṛg-darśana-śaktyoḥ* =

(i) दृक्-शक्तेः *dṛg-śakteḥ* = द्रष्टुः, पुरुषस्य, चेतनतत्त्वस्य of the life-principle

(ii) च *cha* = and

(iii) दर्शन-शक्तेः *darśana-śakteḥ* = बुद्धेः, अचेतनतत्त्वस्य of material-principle

iv) च *cha* = and

v) एकात्मता इव *ekātmatā iva* = एकरूपत्वम् इव भासः the delusion of indifference

vi) 'अस्मिता' *'asmitā'*

vii) इति उच्यते *iti uchyate* = is known as, is called as

📖 **The delusion of indifference between life-principle and material-principle is called as *'asmitā.'* (illusion of indifference).**

✍ Comments : *Asmita* is delusion of indifference. Indifference between life and material principles.

रागः ।

rāgaḥ

15. Attachment

2.7 सुखानुशयी रागः ।

sukhānuśayī rāgaḥ *(sukhā-nuśayī rāgaḥ)*

(o) सुख–अनुशयी *sukhā-nuśayī* =

(i) सुखस्य *sukhasya* = निवृत्तेः, शान्तेः of happiness

(ii) प्रतीतेः *pratiteḥ* = of the conviction, apprehension, fixed belief

(iii) पार्श्वे *parshve* = behind, in the background

(iv) स्थिता *sthitā* = situated

(v) आसक्तिः *asaktiḥ* = the attachment

(vi) 'रागः' *'rāga'*

(vii) इति उच्यते *iti uchyate* = is known as, is called as

📖 **The attachment, situated behind the conviction of happiness, is called as *'rāga.'* (attachment)**

✍ Comments : *Raga* is attachment, Gita (2:56). It gives false impression of happiness.

द्वेषः ।

dveṣaḥ

16. Hatred

2.8 दुःखानुशयी द्वेषः ।

duḥkhānuśayī dveṣaḥ *(duḥkhā-nuśayī dveṣaḥ)*

(o) दुःख–अनुशयी *duḥkhā-nuśayī* =

(i) दुःखस्य *duḥkhasya* = अशान्तेः of pain

(ii) क्लेशस्य *kleshasya* = of affliction

(iii) पार्श्वे *pārshve* = behind

(iv) स्थिता *sthitā* = situated

(v) कुत्सा *kutsā* = hatred, dislike

(vi) 'द्वेषः' *'dveṣaḥ'*

(vii) इति उच्यते *iti uchyate* = is known as, is called as

📖 **The hatred situated behind the affliction of pain is called as *'dveṣaḥ.'***

✍ Comments : *dvesha* afflicts pain.

अभिनिवेषः ।

abhiniveṣaḥ

17. Fear of Death

2.9 स्वरसवाही विदुषोऽपि तथारूढोऽभिनिवेशः ।

svarasavāhī viduṣo'pi tathārūḍho'bhiniveśaḥ

(sva-rasa-vāhī viduṣo-'pi tathā-rūḍho-bhiniveśaḥ)

(o) स्व-रस-वाही *sva-rasa-vāhī* =

(i) परम्परागत: *paramparāgataḥ* = the inherent

(o) विदुषः-अपि-तथा-रूढः *viduṣaḥ-api tathā-rūḍhaḥ* =

(ii) विदुषेषु *viduṣeshu* = विद्वत्सु, विद्वज्जनेषु in the wise people

(iii) अपि *api* = also

(iv) रूढः *rūḍhaḥ* = विद्यमानः that exist

(v) यः मृत्योः भयस्य क्लेशः वर्तते *yaḥ mṛtyoḥ bhayasya kleśḥa vartate* = affliction of the fear of death that exists

(vi) सः *saḥ* = that

(vii) 'अभिनिवेशः' *'abhiniveśaḥ'*

(viii) इति उच्यते *iti uchyate* = is known as, is called as

📖 **The inherent affliction of fear of death that exists in wise people also, is called as *'abhiniveśaḥ.'***

✍ Comments : The fear of death is *abhinivesha.*

2.10 ते प्रतिप्रसवहेयाः सूक्ष्माः ।

te pratiprasavaheyāḥ sūkṣmāḥ *(te prati-prasava-heyāḥ sūkṣmāḥ)*

(i) सूक्ष्माः = गुढाः, तनुविरलाः, श्लक्ष्णाः, स्तोकाः subtle, inherent

(ii) ते = ते क्लेशाः = those hurdles

(iii) प्रति-प्रसव-हेयाः = निर्बिजया समाधिना, चित्तनिग्रहास्त्रेण with the weapon of self-control

(iv) हेया heyā = नाशनीया should be terminated

📖 **Those inherent hurdles should be terminated with the weapon of self-control.**

✍ Comments : Self control is a weapon. It wards off inherent hurdles.

2.11 ध्यानहेयास्तद्वृत्तयः ।

dhyānaheyāstadvṛttayaḥ *(dhyāna-heyāstad-vṛttayaḥ)*

(o) तद्-वृत्तयः *tad-vṛttayaḥ* =

(i) तेषां *tesham* = क्लेषाणाम् of those inherent afflictions

(ii) वृत्तयः *vṛttayaḥ* = अवस्थाः, चित्तावस्थाः states of mind

(o) ध्यान-हेयाः *dhyāna-heyāḥ* =

(iii) ध्यानेन *dhyānena* = ध्यानास्त्रेण with the weapon of contemplation

(iv) हेयाः *heyāḥ* = नाशनीयाः should be terminated

📖 **Those inherent afflictions of states of mind, should be terminated with the weapon of contemplation.**

✍ Comments : Contemplation is a weapon. It removes afflictions of mind.

क्लेशमूलः ।

kleśamūlaḥ

18. The Root of afflictions

2.12 क्लेशमूलः कर्माशयो दृष्टादृष्टजन्मवेदनीयः ।

kleśamūlaḥ karmāśayo dṛṣṭādṛṣṭajanmavedanīyaḥ

(kleśa-mūlaḥ karmāśayo dṛṣṭādṛṣṭa-janma-vedanīyaḥ)

(o) क्लेशमूल: *kleśa-mūlaḥ* =

(i) क्लेश *kleśaḥ* = उपरोक्ता: पञ्च क्लेशा: the above mentioned five afflictions

(ii) मूलानि *mūlāni* = roots

(iii) कर्माशय: *karmāśayaḥ* = कर्मणां समाहारस्य host of karmas

(o) दृष्ट-अदृष्ट-जन्म-वेदनीयम् *dṛṣṭādṛṣṭa-janma-vedanīyam* =

(iv) दृष्टे *dṛṣṭe* = वर्तमाने, गोचरे in visible, tangible, present, animate

(v) अदृष्टे *adṛṣṭe* = अवर्तमाने, अविद्यमाने, अगोचरे in invisible, intangible, inanimate

(vi) जन्मनि *janmani* = पुनर्जन्मनि in rebirth

(vii) 'भोग:' *'bhogaḥ,'* = to be experienced in

(viii) इति वेदनीयं *iti vedanīyam* = ज्ञातव्यम्, ज्ञेयम् should be considered as

The host of *karmas* are the roots, of the above mentioned five afflictions. They are to be experienced in animate and inanimate births.

Comments : *Karmas* are responsible for (i) perversion of mind, (ii) illusion of indifference, (iii) attachment, (iv) hatred and (v) longing to stay alive.

2.13 सति मूले तद्विपाको जात्यायुर्भोगाः ।

sati mule tadvipako jātyāyurbhogāḥ

(sati mule tad-vipako jātyāyur-bhogāḥ)

(i) मूले-सति *mule -sati* = मूलस्य विद्यतायाम् while in the existence of these roots

(o) तत्-विपाक: *tat-vipakaḥ* =

(ii) तत् *tat* = तेषां कर्मणाम् of the karmas

(iii) विपाक: *vipakaḥ* = परिणाम:, कर्मफलम् result

(o) जाति-आयु-भोगा: *jātyāyur-bhogāḥ* =

(iv) जाति *jāti* = जाति पुनर्जन्म re-birtth

(v) आयु: *āyuḥ* = जीवनम्, जीवनकाल: the life span

(vi) भोग: *bhogāḥ* = अनुभव: the experience

(viii) भवति *bhavati* = is

📖 **While, in the existence of these roots of the *karmas,* the result is the experience of the life span and rebirth.**

✍ Comments : The *karma* is responsible for rebirth. Gita (8:3).

2.14 ते ह्लादपरितापफला: पुण्यापुण्यहेतुत्वात् ।

te lhādaparitāpafalāḥ puṇyāpuṇyahetutvāt

(te lhāda-paritāpa-falāḥ puṇyāpuṇya-hetutvāt)

(i) ते *te* = तौ पुनर्जन्मन: आयुस: च भोगौ those experiences of rebirth and life span

(o) ह्लाद-परिताप-फला: *lhāda-paritāpa-falāḥ* =

(ii) ह्लाद: *lhādaḥ* = हर्ष:, आमोद:, सुखम् happiness

(ii) परिताप: *a-paritāpaḥ* = शोक:, दु:खम् unhappiness

(iii) आदिनां फला: *ādi falāḥ* = फलदायका: are the givers of the fruits

(iv) सन्ति *santi* = are

(o) पुण्य-अपुण्य-हेतुत्वात् *puṇyāpuṇya-hetutvāt* =

(v) अत: *ataḥ* = therefore

(vi) तेषां *tesham* = their

(vii) पुण्यकर्म च पापकर्म च *puṇya-karma cha pāp-karma cha* = the good deeds and the bad deeds

(viii) द्वेऽपि *dve-pi* = both

(ix) कारणौ *kāran,au* = their causes

(x) स्त: *staḥ* = are

📖 **Those experiences of (i) birth, (ii) life span and (iii) rebirth are the givers of** the fruits of happiness and unhappiness. Therefore, their causes are both the good deeds and the bad deeds.

✍ Comments : The good deeds (*punya*) and bad deeds (*papa*) are the givers of happiness and unhappiness in lives.

दुःखम् ।
duḥkham
19. Unhappiness

2.15 परिणामतापसंस्कारदुःखैर्गुणवृत्तिविरोधाच्च दुःखमेव सर्वं विवेकिनः ।

pariṇāmatāpsaṁskāraduḥkhairguṇavṛttivirodhāccá duḥkhameva sarvam vivikinaḥ

(pariṇāma-tāp-saṁskāra-duḥkhair-guṇa-vṛtti-virodhāc-ća duḥkham-eva sarvam vivikinaḥ)

(o) परिणाम–ताप–संस्कार–दुःखैः *pariṇāma-tāp-saṁskāra-duḥkhaiḥ* =

(i) परिणामस्य दुःखेन *pariṇāmasya duḥkhena* = due to unhappiness as a result of these afflictions

(ii) तापस्य दुःखेन *tāpasya duḥkhena* = and due to unhappiness as a result of anguish

(iii) संस्कारस्य दुःखेन *saṁskārasya duḥkhena* = as a result of previous unhappy impression

(iv) च *cha* = and

(o) गुण–वृत्ति–विरोधात् *vṛtti-virodhāċ* =

(v) गुणानां च वृत्तिनां च परस्पराभ्यां *guṇānām cha vṛttinām cha parasparābhyām* = from both the attributes and the mind sets

(vi) विरोधात् *virodhāt* = असङ्गत्याः, विसंवादात् विपरितातायाः, व्याघातात् by the opposition

(vii) विवेकिनः *vivikinaḥ* = विद्वते for the wise person

(viii) दुःखम् इव *duḥkham iva* = like an unhappiness

(ix) एव *eva* = just, only

(x) सन्ति *santi* = are

📖 **Due to unhappiness as a result of these afflictions : (i) anguish and (ii) previous unhappy impression, and from these two (iii) the opposition by the attributes and (iv) the opposition by the mind sets, for the wise person they all are just like one unhappiness.**

✍ Comments : All afflictions are collectively one unhappiness.

2.16 हेयं दुःखमनागतम् ।

heyam duḥkhamanāgatam *(heyam duḥkham-anāgatam)*

(i) अन्–आगतम् *an-āgatam* = न आगतम्, यत् आगमिष्यति तत् the one that has not yet come up on

(ii) दुःखं *duḥkham* = the pain

(iii) हेयम् *heyam* = हन्तव्यम्, हननीयम्, नाशितव्यम् should be prevented before it comes

📖 **The pain that has not yet come up on, should be prevented before it comes.**

✍ Comments : Pain should be prevented.

2.17 द्रष्टृदृश्ययोः संयोगो हेयहेतुः ।

draṣṭṛdṛśyayoḥ saṁyogo heyahetuḥ *(draṣṭṛ-dṛśyayoḥ saṁyogo heya-hetuḥ)*

(o) द्रष्टृ–दृश्ययोः *draṣṭṛ-dṛśyayoḥ* =

(i) द्रष्टुः *draṣṭuḥ* = पश्यतः of the beholder

(ii) च *cha* = and

(iii) दृश्यस्य *dṛśyasya* = दृश्यमानस्य to be seen, the thing that is visible, the perceptible world

(iv) च *cha* = and

(v) संयोगः *samyogaḥ* = सम्बन्धः, संश्लेशः, सम्पर्कः, योगः the bondage, union

(o) हेय-हेतुः *heya-hetuḥ* =

(vi) हेयः *heyaḥ* = नाशनीयस्य for that on coming pain which is to be terminated

(vii) हेतुः *hetuḥ* = कारणम्, उद्देशः, निमित्तम्, प्रयोजनम् the cause

(viii) अस्ति *asti* = is

📖 **The union of 'beholder' and 'the perceptible' is the cause for that on-coming pain which is to be terminated.**

✍ Comments : Union of the beholder and the perceptible is the cause of pain.

दृश्यम् ।

dṛśyam

20. The preceptible world

2.18 प्रकाशक्रियास्थितिशीलं भूतेन्द्रियात्मकं भोगापवर्गार्थं दृश्यम् ।

prakāśakriyāsthitiśīlam bhūtendriyātmakam

bhogāpavargārtham dṛśyam

(prakāśa-kriyāsthiti-śīlam bhūte-ndriyatmakam bhogāpavargārtham dṛśyam)

(o) प्रकाश-क्रिया-स्थिति-शीलम् *prakāśa-kriyāsthiti-śīlam* =

(ii) प्रकाश *prakāśa* = सत्-गुणः sat-guṇaḥ

(ii) क्रिया *kriyā* = रजोगुणः rajo-guṇaḥ

(iv) स्थिति *sthitiḥ* = तमोगुणः tamo-guṇaḥ

(v) शीलं *śīlam* = शीलं यस्य धर्मः, गुणः स्वभावः अस्ति तत् of which nature is that

(vi) च *cha* = and

(o) भूत-इन्द्रियात्मकम् *bhūta-indriyatmakam* =

(vii) भूतानि *bhūtāni* = the beings

(viii) इन्द्रियाणि च *indriyāṇi cha* = with their eleven organs

(ix) यस्य गोचरं स्वरूपम् अस्ति *yasya gocharam svarūpam asti* = which has visible nature

(x) तत् *tat* = that

(xi) भोगापवर्गार्थम् *bhogāpavargārtham* = यस्य च अर्थः भोगः अस्ति of which purpose is experience

(xii) 'दृश्यम्' *'dṛśyam'* = dṛśyam

(xiii) इति उच्यते *iti uchyate* = is known as, is called as

That, visible nature (i) which is caused by *sat-guṇaḥ, rajo-guṇaḥ* and *tamo-guṇaḥ* and (ii) with which the beings experience things with their eleven organs, is called as *'dṛśyam.'*

Comments : The visible being, composed of three *gunas* and eleven organs, is *drashya.*

The three *gunas* are *sat, rajas* and *tamas* (Gita 14:5). The eleven organs are (i) five work organs, (ii) five sense organs and (iii) the mind. The five work organs are (i) hands, (ii) legs, (iii) mouth, (iv) organ of excretion, () organ of propagation (Gita 3:6). The five sense organs are (i) ears, (ii) eyes, (iii) tongue (iv) nose and (v) skin. and the eleventh organ is the mind (Gita 15:7).

गुणाः ।

guṇāḥ

21. Attributes

2.19 विशेषाविशेषलिङ्गमात्रालिङ्गानि गुणपर्वाणि ।

viśeṣāviśeṣaliṅgamātrāliṅgāni guṇaparvāṇi

(viśeṣāviśeṣa-liṅga-mātrāliṅgāni guṇa-parvāṇi)

(o) विशेष-अविशेष-लिङ्ग-मात्र-अलिङ्गानि *viśeṣāviśeṣa-liṅga-mātrāliṅgāni* =

(i) विशेष *viśeṣa* = पृथ्वयप्तेजस्वायवाकाशानि पञ्च-महाभूतानि त्वक्रसनाचक्षुस्कर्णघ्राणानि पञ्च-ज्ञानेन्द्रियाणि वाक्पाणिपादपायूपस्थानि पञ्च-कर्मेन्द्रियाणि षोडषं च मनः the five primary elements namely earth, water, fire, wind and sky; the five sense organs namely skin, tongue, eyes, ears and nose; five motor organs namely mouth, hands, legs, organ of reproduction and excretion; and the sixteenth, mind

(ii) अविशेष *aviśeṣa* = स्पर्शशब्दरूपरसगन्धाः पञ्च-तन्मात्राः the five subtle elements namely touch, speech, sight, taste and smell

(iii) लिङ्ग-मात्रं *liṅga-mātram* = बुद्धिः the cognition

(iv) अलिङ्गम् *āliṅgam* = मूल-प्रकृतिः, सद्ररजस्तमस्त्रिगुणानां सामान्यावस्था the normal balance of the three attributes namely sat, rajas and tamas

(v) इति गुण-पर्वाणि *iti guṇa-parvāṇi* = गुण-स्थितयः the four states in which are the three guṇa attributes

(vi) दृश्यानि *dṛśyāni* = preceptible

(vii) सन्ति *santi* = are

(i) The group of five primary elements namely : earth, water, fire, wind and sky; the five sense organs namely : skin, tongue, eyes, ears and nose; and five motor organs namely : mouth, hands, legs, organ of reproduction and excretion; and sixteenth : the mind; (ii) the five subtle elements namely : touch, speech, sight, taste and smell; (iii) the cognition; and (iv) the normal balance of the three attributes namely : *sat, rajas* and *tamas* - are the four states in which the three attributes are perceptible.

दृष्टा ।

dṛṣṭā

22. Beholder

2.20 द्रष्टा दृशिमात्रः शुद्धोऽपि प्रत्ययानुपश्यः ।

draṣṭā dṛśimātraḥ śuddho'pi pratyānupaśyaḥ

(draṣṭā dṛśi-mātraḥ śuddho'pi pratyā-nupaśyaḥ)

(i) दृशि–मात्र: *dṛśi-mātraḥ* = चेतनतत्त्वं, आत्मतत्त्वम् the life principle that is called atmā

(ii) शुद्ध: *śuddhaḥ* = निर्विकार:, अक्षर:, अक्षय:, अव्यय: eternal

(iii) अपि *api* = अस्ति तथापि even though

(iv) प्रत्यय–अनुपश्य: *pratyā-nupaśyaḥ* = बुद्धे: संसर्गेण by his association with cognition

(v) वृत्ति: अनुपश्यति *vṛttiḥ anupaśyaṭi* = he behaves accordingly

(vi) अत: *ataḥ* = and therefore

(vii) स: *saḥ* = he

(viii) 'दृष्टा' *'dṛṣṭā,'* = the beholder

(ix) इति उच्यते *iti uchyate* = is known as, is called as

📖 **The life principle that is called *atmā,* even though eternal, by his association with cognition he behaves accordingly, and therefore, he is called as *'dṛṣṭā'* (beholder).**

✍ Comments : The *ātmā* is *drashta,* the beholder.

दृश्यम् ।

dṛśyam

23. Beheld

2.21 तदर्थ एव दृश्यस्यात्मा ।

tadartha eva dṛśyasyātmā *(tad-artha eva dṛśyasy-ātmā)*

(i) दृश्यस्य *dṛśyasya* = द्रष्टा यत् अवलोकति, पश्यति, आलोचति, लक्षति, ईक्षति, विक्षति, अन्विष्यति, अनुभवति तत् = whatever the beholder ātmā beholds

(ii) तस्य *tasya* = its

(iii) आत्मा *ātmā* = अन्तरङ्गम्, अन्त:स्वरूपम् inward nature

(iv) तदर्थः एव *tad-artha eva* = तस्मै द्रष्ट्रे एव अस्ति is for the purpose of the beholder ātmā only

📖 **Whatever the beholder *ātmā* beholds is dṛṣya. The inward nature of the beheld is for the purpose of the beholder *ātmā* only.**

✍ Comments : Whatever the *atma* beholds is *drashya,* the beheld.

2.22 कृतार्थं प्रति नष्टमप्यनष्टं तदन्यसाधारणत्वात् ।

kṛtārtham prati naṣṭamapyanaṣṭam tadnyasādhāraṇatvāt

(kṛtārtham prati naṣṭam-apyanaṣṭam tadnya-sādhāraṇatvāt)

(o) कृतार्थं प्रति *kṛtārtham prati* =

(ii) यः कृतकार्यः *yaḥ kṛtaakāryaḥ* = सफलः, सिद्धार्थः whose the purpose is served

(iii) अस्ति *asti* = is,

(iv) तस्मै *tasmai* = for him

(vi) निष्प्रयोजनाय *niṣprayojanāya* = for having no purpose any more

(vii) नष्टम् *naṣṭam* = पुनः कार्यस्य प्रयोजनं न विद्यते तम्, यस्य कार्यं न विद्यते तम् for that there is no function

(viii) अपि = च and

(ix) अनष्टम् *anaṣṭam* = यः अकृतार्थः, असफलः, असिद्धार्थः, यस्य कार्यस्य प्रयोजनं विद्यते तम् the function of which purpose is not yet served

(x) तत् *tat* = तत् प्रकृतेः प्रयोजनम् that purpose of the inward nature

(xi) अन्य-साधारणत्वात् *anyasādhāraṇatvāt* = कृतार्थ-अकृतार्थयोः served and not-served

(xii) समानम् एव अस्ति *samanam eva asti* = are both same.

📖 **For that, whose the purpose is served, there is no function. And, whose purpose is not yet served, there is function. Because, that purpose of inward nature served and not-served are both same.**

✍ Comments : The purpose of the inward nature is always served.

संयोगः ।

saṁyogaḥ

24. Union

2.23 स्वस्वामिशक्त्योः स्वरूपोपलब्धिहेतुः संयोगः ।

svasvāmiśaktyoḥ svarūpopalabdhihetuḥ saṁyogaḥ

(sva-svāmi-śaktyoḥ sva-rūpo-palabdhi-hetuḥ saṁyogaḥ)

(o) स्व-स्वामिशक्त्योः *sva-svāmi-śaktyoḥ* =

(i) स्व-शक्तेः *sva-śakteḥ* = स्व-प्रकृतेः, स्व-भावस्य of your physical principle (and)

(ii) स्वामिशक्तेः *svāmi-śakteḥ* = पुरुषस्य, आत्मतत्त्वस्य of the life principle, of the ātmā

(o) स्वरूप-उपलब्धि-हेतुः *sva-rūpo-palabdhi-hetuḥ* =

(iii) स्वरूपस्य *sva-rūp* = प्रकृतेः, स्वभावस्य nature of

(iv) उपलब्धेः *upalabdheḥ* = प्राप्तेः, उपपत्तेः attainment, coming together of

(v) हेतुः *hetuḥ* = उद्देशः, प्रयोजनम्, कारणम् purpose

(vi) 'संयोगः' 'saṁyogaḥ'

(vii) इति उच्यते *iti uchyate* = is known as, is called as

📖 **Coming together of the purpose of your physical principle and the *ātmā* is called as *'saṁyogaḥ'* (union).**

✍ Comments : Coming together of the body and *atma* is *samyoga.*

अविद्या ।

avidyā

25. Perversion of mind

2.24 तस्य हेतुरविद्या ।

tasya heturavidyā *(tasya hetur-avidyā)*

(i) तस्य *tasya* = तस्य संयोगस्य for that saṁyoga, that coming to gether, that union

(ii) हेतुः *hetuḥ* = उद्देशः, प्रयोजनम्, कारणम् the reason

(iii) 'अविद्या' 'avidyā'

(iv) एव भवति *eva bhavati* = is

📖 ***Avidyā* is the reason for that *saṁyoga.***

✍ Comments : *Avidya* causes the union of the body and the *atma.*

हानम् कैवल्यम् च ।

hānam kaivalyam ća

26. Future Pains and Liberation

2.25 तदभावात्संयोगाभावो हानं तद्दृशेः कैवल्यम् ।

tadabhāvātsaṁyogābhavo hānam taddṛśeḥ kaivalyam

(tad-abhāvāt-saṁyogā-bhavo hānam tad-dṛśeḥ kaivalyam)

(o) तत्-अभावात् *tad-abhāvāt* =

(i) तस्याः *tasyāḥ* = of that

(ii) अविद्यायाः *avidyāyāḥ* = perversion of mind

(iii) अभावात् *abhāvāt* = अविद्यमानतायाः with the absence

(iv) संयोग-अभावः *saṁyog-abhāvaḥ* = संयोगः न विद्यते saṁyoga does not take place

(v) ततः *tataḥ* = and from that

(vi) हानम् *hānam* = भविष्याणां दुःखानां अभावः non-existence of future pains

(vii) अपि च भवति *api cha bhavati* = also occurs

(viii) तत् *tat* = ततः सः = therefore that

(ix) असंयोगः एव *a saṁyogaḥ eva* = non-saṁyoga, non-union, not coming together

(x) दृशेः *dṛśeḥ* = चेतनस्य आत्मनः of the living principle ātmā

(xi) 'कैवल्यम्' *kaivalyam* = liberation

(xi) इति उच्यते *iti uchyate* = is known as, is called as

📖 **With the absence of that perversion of mind, *saṁyoga* does not take place. And from that, non-existence of future pains also occurs. Therefore, that not coming together of the living principle *ātmā* (with your physical principle), is called as *'kaivalyam.'* (liberation)**

✍ Comments : *Kaivalya* is final liberation. It is also called *mokshya* or *brahma-nirvana* (Gita 2.72).

विवेकः ।

vivekaḥ

27. Discernment

2.26 विवेकख्यातिरविप्लवा हानोपायः ।

vivekakhyātiraviplavā hānopāyaḥ

(viveka-khyātir-aviplavā hano-pāyaḥ)

(i) अ-विप्लवा *aviplavā* = अनघा, निष्कलङ्का, निर्विघ्ना untainted

(o) विवेक-ख्यातिः *viveka-khyātiḥ* =

(ii) यस्य ख्यातिः *yasya-khyātiḥ* = संज्ञा, नाम of which the designation is ...

(iii) 'विवेकः' *'vivekaḥ,* = discernment

(iv) इति अस्ति *iti asti* = is

(v) तत् 'ज्ञानम्' *tat jñānam* = that comprehension

(vi) इति मन्तव्यम् *iti mantavyam* = should also be understood as

(vii) हान-उपाय: *hana upāyaḥ* =

(viii) उपरोक्तस्य *uparoktasya* = of the above mentioned see 2.25 above

(ix) हानस्य *hanasya* = भविष्याणां दुःखानां अभावस्य for the absence of future pains

(x) उपाय: *upāyaḥ* = युक्तिः, साधनम्, करणम्, उपकरणम्, सामग्री the remedy

(xi) अपि वर्तते *api vartate* = is also

📖 **That untrained, of which the designation is *'vivekaḥ,'* (discernment), should also be understood as comprehension. That is also the remedy for the above mentioned absence of future pains**

✍ Comments : *Viveka* is comprehension. *Viveka* prevents pains. It is the *Ritambhara* meditation.

प्रज्ञा ।

prajñā

28. Cognition

2.27 तस्य सप्तधा प्रान्तभूमिः प्रज्ञा ।

tasyasaptadhā prāntabhūmiḥ prajñā

(tasyasaptadhā prānta-bhūmiḥ prajñā)

(i) तस्य *tasya* = येन विवेकज्ञानं प्राप्तं तस्य that by which discernment is achieved

(ii) सप्तधा *saptadhā* = सप्तविधा sevenfold

(iii) प्रान्तभूमिः *prānta-bhūmiḥ* = परिक्षेपः, ज्ञानवलयः aura

(iv) 'प्रज्ञा' *prajñā* = बुद्धिः 'prajñā,' cognition

(v) इति उच्यते *iti uchyate* = is known as, is called as

📖 **That discernment, by which sevenfold aura is achieved, is called as *'prajñā'***

(cognition).

✍ Comments : *Prajña* is aura.

2.28 योगाङ्गानुष्ठानादशुद्धिक्षये ज्ञानदीप्तिराविवेकख्यातेः ।

yogāṅgānuṣṭhānādaśuddhikṣaye jñānadīptirāvivekakhyāteḥ

(yogāṅgānuṣṭhānād-aśuddhi-kṣaye jñāna-dīptir-āviveka-khyāteḥ)

(o) योग-अङ्ग-अनुष्ठानात् *yogāṅgānuṣṭhānāt*

(i) योगस्य *yogasya* = of yoga

(ii) अष्ट-अङ्गानाम् *aṣṭa- aṅgānām* = the eight components

(iii) अनुष्ठानात् *anuṣṭhānāt* = आचरणात्, स-विधि-संपादनात् from accomplishment

(iv) अशुद्धि-क्षये *aśuddhi-kṣaye* = अशुद्धेः, त्रुटेः, भ्रान्तेः, दोषस्य of the pollution, contamination

(v) क्षये *kṣaye* = ह्रासात्, अपचयात्, अन्तात्, नाशात् as a result of removal of

(vi) ज्ञानदीप्तिः *jñāna-dīptiḥ* = ज्ञानप्रकाशः, आत्मनः स्वरूपं मनसः च इन्द्रियेभ्यः च भिन्नम् अस्ति इति ज्ञानम् the light of knowledge that the nature of ātma is different than the natures of mind and organs

(o) आ-विवेक-ख्यातेः *āviveka-khyāteḥ* =

(vii) स-विचारः प्रत्यक्ष-रूपेण *saḥ vichāraḥ pratyakṣa rūpeṇa* = in the light clearly

(viii) दृश्यते *dṛśyate* = appears, reveals

📖 **From accomplishment of the eight components of *yoga* (2.29↑), as a result of removal of pollution, the light of knowledge reveals clearly that the nature of *ātma* is different than the natures of mind and organs.**

✍ Comments : The nature of *atma* is different than the natures ten organs and the mind.

योगाङ्गाः ।

yogāṅgāḥ

29. Component of Yoga

2.29 यमनियमासनप्राणायामप्रत्याहारधारणाध्यानसमाधयोऽष्टावङ्गानि ।

yamaniyamāsanaprāṇāyāmapartyāhāradhāraṇādhyāna-samādhayo'ṣṭāvaṅgāni

(yama-niyamāsana-prāṇāyāma-partyāhāra-dhāraṇādhyāna-samādhayo-'ṣṭāv-aṅgāni)

(o) यम-नियम-आसन-प्राणायम-प्रत्याहार-धारणा-ध्यान-समाधय: *yama-niyamāsana-prāṇāyāma- partyāhāra-dhāraṇādhyāna-samādhayaḥ* =

(i) यम: *yamaḥ* = इन्द्रिय-निग्रहः, मनोनिग्रहः, अहिंसा-सत्य-अस्तेय-ब्रह्मचर्य-अपरिग्रहः-धर्मपालनम् self control

(ii) नियमः *niyamaḥ* = इन्द्रियाणां मनसः च सङ्कल्पः, नियन्त्रणम्, प्रतिबन्धः, निदेशः observance

(iii) आसनं *āsanam* = स्थितिः, उपवेशन-प्रकारः posture

(iv) प्राणायमः *prāṇāyāmaḥ* = श्वास-निःश्चास-गति-निरोधः breath control

(v) प्रत्याहारः *partyāhāraḥ* = उपादानम्, अल्पेन बहुनां ग्रहणम् withholding

(vi) धारणा *dhāraṇā* = ध्येये चित्तस्य स्थिरबन्धनम् focus on aim

(vii) ध्यानम् *dhyānam* = ऐकाग्र्यम्, एकावधानम् concentration

(viii) समाधिः *samādhiḥ* = अन्तर्ध्यानम्, समाधानम्, अनन्यमनस्कता, निःस्तब्धता meditation

(ix) अष्ट *aṣṭa* = एतानि अष्ट these eight, eight

(x) अङ्गानि *aṅgāni* = योगस्य अङ्गानि, प्रतीकाः, अंशाः, भागाः, अवयवाः components

(xi) सन्ति *santi* = are

📖 **(i) Self control, (ii) observance, (iii) posture, (iv) breath control, (v) withholding, (vi) focus on aim (vii) concentration and (viii) meditation are eight components of *yoga*.**

✍ Comments : Given below are the descriptions of the eight components of yoga.

यमाः ।

yamāḥ

30. Self-controls

2.30 अहिंसासत्यास्तेयब्रह्मचर्यापरिग्रहाः यमाः ।

ahiṁsāsatyāsteyabrahmacharyāparigrahāḥ yamāḥ

(ahiṁsā-satyāsteya-brahmacharyā-parigrahāḥ yamāḥ)

(o) अहिंसा-सत्य-अस्तेय-ब्रह्मचर्य-अपरिग्रहाः *ahiṁsā-satyāsteya-brahmacharyā-parigrahāḥ* =

(i) अहिंसा *ahiṁsā* = हत्या-अपकार-द्रोह-वैरादिनां त्यागः non-violence through deeds, words and thought by forsaking of all forms of killing, harm, treachery and enmity

(ii) सत्यं *satyam* = ऋतम्, तथ्यम्, तत्त्वम्, यथार्थम्, अकृत्रिमम् truthfulness

(iii) अस्तेयं *asteyam* = अचौर्यम्, न पर-द्रव्य-ग्रहणम् non-stealing

(iv) ब्रह्मचर्यं *brahmacharyam-* = अष्टाङ्ग-मैथुन-प्रतिषेधः, ऊर्ध्व-रेतस्त्वम्, वीर्यरक्षा sexual restraint

(v) अपरिग्रहः *aparigrahāḥ* = असञ्चयनम् non-hoarding

(vi) इति 'यमाः' *iti 'yamāḥ'* = self-controls

(vii) सन्ति *santi* = are, are five

📖 **(i) Non-violence through deeds, words and thought by forsaking of all forms of killing, harm, treachery and enmity, (ii) truthfulness, (iii) non-stealing, (iv) sexual restraint and (v) non-hoarding are five *yamāḥ,'* (self-controls) .**

✍ Comments : The five components of self control are : (i) non-violence, (ii) truth, (iii) honesty, (iv) abstinence and (iv) non-coveting.

विश्वत्वम् ।

viśvatvam

31. universality

2.31 जातिदेशकालसमयानवच्छिन्नाः सार्वभौमा महाव्रतम् ।

jātideśakālasamayānavacchinnāḥ sārvabhaumā mahāvratam

(jāti-deśa-kāla-samayān-avacchinnāḥ sārva-bhaumā mahā-vratam)

(o) जाति–देश–काल–समय–अनवच्छिन्नाः *jāti-deśa-kāla-samayān-avacchinnāḥ* =

(i) जातिः *jātiḥ* = जन्म birth

(ii) देशः *deśaḥ* = स्थानम्, स्थलम् place

(iii) कालः *kālaḥ* = घटि, क्षणः time

(iv) समयः *samayaḥ* = निमित्तम् cause

(v) आदिषु *ādiṣu* = in ... etc.

(vi) अनवच्छिन्नः *avacchinnāḥ* = सीमा–हीनः, असीमः not bound, unrestricted, unhindered, unaffected

(vii) सार्वभौमाः *sārva-bhaumāḥ* = सर्वस्मिन् स्थले–काले–समये universal

(viii) च *cha* = and

(ix) महा–व्रतम् *mahā-vratam* = great austerity

📖 **It is a great universal austerity, unrestricted by birth, place, time, cause, ...etc.**

✍ Comments : Yoga is greatest Universal Austerity for all.

नियमाः ।

niyamāḥ

32. Restraints

2.32 शौचसन्तोषतपःस्वाध्यायेश्वरप्रणिधानि नियमाः ।

saućasantoṣatapaḥsvādhyāyeśvarapraṇidhāni niyamāḥ

(sauća-santoṣa-tapaḥ-svādhyāye-śvara-praṇidhāni niyamāḥ)

(o) शौच-सन्तोष-तपः-स्वाध्याय-ईश्वर-प्रणिधानि *sauća-santoṣa-tapaḥ-svādhyāye-śvara-praṇidhāni* =

(i) शौचं *saućam* = पावित्र्यम्, धार्मिकत्वम्, शुद्धिः purity

(ii) सन्तोषः *santoṣaḥ* = तृप्तिः, तुष्टिः, तोषः, शान्तिः, समाधानम्, वितृष्णा satisfaction, contentment

(iii) तपः *tapaḥ* = स्वधर्मस्य स्वगुणानुसारेण सर्वदा पालनंम् austerity

(iv) स्वाध्यायः *svādhyāyaḥ* = शास्त्राभ्यासः study of scriptures

(v) ईश्वर-प्रणिधानं *iśvara-praṇidhānam* = ईश्वरं प्रति, भगवतः प्रति, भगवन्तं प्रति श्रद्धा, निष्ठा, भक्तिः faith in God

(vi) इति पञ्च *iti pañcha* = five

(vii) 'नियमाः' *'niyamāḥ,'* = observances

(viii) कथ्यन्ते *kathyante* = are called as

📖 **Purity, contentment, austerity, study of scriptures and faith in God are called as five *'niyamāḥ,'* (observances).**

✍ Comments : The *niyamas* are the rules of pure life or the yogic life.

वितर्कः हिंसा लोभः क्रोधः मोहः च ।

vitarkaḥ hiṁsā lobhaḥ krodhaḥ mohaḥ ća

33. Doubt, Violence, Greed, Angerand and Delusion

2.33 वितर्कबाधने प्रतिपक्षभावनम् ।

vitarkabādhane pratipakṣabhāvanam

(vitarka-bādhane prati-pakṣa-bhāvanam)

(i) वितर्क-बाधने *vitarka-bādhane* = वितर्कात् बाधायां, वितर्कः-ऊहः-सन्देहः यदा यम-नियमेषु बाधां करोति तदा if a doubt hinders the self-control and the observances

(o) प्रति-पक्ष-भावनम् *prati-pakṣa-bhāvanam* =

(ii) तदा तस्य वितर्कस्य निवारणार्थाय = remedy for the removal of that doubt

(iii) तत्र स्थितान् दोषान् अवगन्तुं = to understand the obstacles hindering the self control and the observances

(iv) चिन्तनं करणीयम् *ćintanam karanīyam* = one should meditate up on

If a doubt hinders the self-control and the observances, one should meditate up on the remedy to understand the obstacles hindering the self control and the observances for the removal of that doubt.

Comments : Doubt hinders self control. One should meditate on remedy to remove doubt.

दोषाः ।

doṣāḥ

34. Obstacles

2.34 वितर्का हिंसादयः कृतकारितानुमोदिता लोभक्रोधमोहपूर्वका मृदुमध्याधिकमात्रा दुःखाज्ञानानन्तफला इति प्रतिपक्षभावम् ।

vitarkā hiṁsādayaḥ kṛtakāritānumoditā

lobhakrodhamohapūrvakā

mṛdumadhyādhikamātrā duḥkhājñānānantaphalā

iti pratipakṣabhāvam

(vitarkā hiṁsādayaḥ kṛta-kāritāanumoditā lobha-krodha-moha-pūrvakā

mṛdu-madhyādhika-mātrā duḥkhājñānā-nanta-phalā iti prati-pakṣa-bhāvam)

(i) हिंसादय: *hiṁsādayaḥ* = यमस्य च नियमस्य च विरोधी, हिंसका: the hindering to self control and observances such as violence etc.

(ii) भावा: *bhāvāḥ* = emotions

(iii) ये त्रिधा सन्ति *ye tridhā santi* = which are of three types, namely :

(o) कृत-कारित-अनुमोदिता: *kṛta-kāritāanumoditā ḥ* =

(vi) स्वयं कृता: *sva-kṛtāḥ* = self created (and)

(vi) अपरै: कारयिता: *aparaiḥ kāritāḥ* = induced by others (and)

(vii) अपरै: सह अनुमोदिता: इति *aparai saha anumoditāḥ* = instigated by others

(viii) ते त्रिविधा: भावा: *te trividhāḥ bhāvāḥ* = of these three types of sentiments

(o) मृदु-मध्य-अधिक-मात्रा: *mṛdu-madhyādhika-mātrāḥ* =

(x) केचन मृदु *kechan mṛdu* = some are minor

(xi) केचन मध्य *kechan madhya* = मध्यम-परिणाम-कारक some are moderate

(xii) केचन अधिक *kechan adhika* = आत्यन्तिक, अमित some are of severe

(xiii) मात्रा: *matrā* = मात्राया: of influence

(xiv) भवन्ति *bhavanti* = are

(o) दु:ख-अज्ञान-अनन्त-फला: *duḥkhājñānā-nanta-phalāḥ* =

(xvi) ते सर्वे *te sarve* = they all

(xvii) अनन्तं दु:खं *anantam duḥkham* = endless anguish

(xviii) च अज्ञानं *cha ajñānam* = perversion

(xix) फलरूपेण *phala-rupeṇa* = in the form of fruit, result

(xx) ददति *dadati* = give

(xxi) इति *iti* = एतानि these

(xxii) प्रति-पक्ष-भावा: *prati-pakṣa-bhāvāḥ* = प्रतिपक्षस्य दोषा: external obstacles

(xxiii) बोधनीया: *bodhanīyāḥ* = are to be considered as

🕮 The hindering emotions to self control and observances such as violence etc.

which are of three types, namely (i) self created, (ii) induced by others and (iii) instigated by others. Of these three types of sentiments, some are minor, some are moderate and some are of severe influence. They all give endless anguish and perversion in the form of result. These are to be considered as external *'doṣāḥ'* (obstacles).

✍ Comments : *Dosha* is an emotion that hinders self control. *Dosha* gives anguish and perversion.

अहिंसा मैत्र्यम् अस्तेयम् ब्रह्मचर्यम् च ।

ahim̃sā maitryam asteyam btahmacharyam ća

35. non-violence, brotherhood, non-stealing and celibacy

2.35 अहिंसाप्रतिष्ठायां तत्सन्निधौ वैरत्यागः ।

ahimsāpratiṣṭhāyām tatsannidhau vairatyāgaḥ

(ahimsā-pratiṣṭhāyām tat-sannidhau vaira-tyāgaḥ)

(o) अहिंसा-प्रतिष्ठायाम् *ahimsā-pratiṣṭhāyām* =

(i) उपरोक्तायाः चतुर्विधायाः अहिंसायाः *uparoktāyāḥ chaturvidhāyāḥ ahim̃sāyāḥ* = of above mentioned four-way non-violence through deeds, words and thought by forsaking of all forms of killing, harm, treachery and enmity

(ii) भावना *bhāvanā* = the feeling

(iii) मनसि यदा *yadā manasi* = when in the mind

(iv) दृढा भवति *dṛḍhā bhavati* = becomes firm

(v) तदा *tadā* = then

(vi) तत्-सन्निधौ *tasya sannidhau* = तस्य योगिनः प्रति towards that yogī

(vii) सर्वाणि भूतानि *sarvāṇi bhūtāni* = all beings

(viii) वैर त्यागः *vaira-tyāgaḥ* = वैरभावं त्यजन्ति give up enmity

(ix) इत्युक्ते *ityukte* = in other words

(x) न कोऽपि वैरभावं करोति *na kopi vaira bhāvam karoti* = no one has enmity to him

📖 **When in the mind of *yogī* the feeling of above mentioned three-way non-violence through (i) deeds, (ii) words and (iii) thought, by forsaking of all forms of killing, harm, treachery and enmity : becomes firm, then no one has enmity towards that *yogī*.**

✍ Comments : A *yogi* who has no *dosha*, has no enemies.

सत्यप्रतिष्ठा ।

satyapratiṣṭhā

36. Truthfulness

2.36 सत्यप्रतिष्ठायां क्रियाफलाश्रयत्वम् ।

satyapratiṣṭhāyām kiryāphalāśrayatvam

(satya-pratiṣṭhāyām kiryā-phalāśrayatvam)

(o) सत्य-प्रतिष्ठायाम् *satya-pratiṣṭhāyām* =

(i) यदा *yadā* = when

(ii) योगिन: *yoginaḥ* = of the yogi

(iii) सत्यं प्रति *satyam-prati* = towards truth

(iv) दृढा भावना *dṛḍha bhāvanā* = firm resolve

(v) भवति *bhavati* = becomes

(vi) तदा *tadā* = then

(o) क्रिया-फल-आश्रयत्वम् *kiryā-phalāśrayatvam* =

(vii) तस्य योगिन: *tasya yoginaḥ* = of that yogī

viii) कर्माणि *karmāni* = the deeds

(ix) फलं प्रति *phalam prati* = towards the result

(x) इतरेषां आश्रयः *itareṣām āśrayaḥ* = पर-उद्देशः, परलाभः, परमार्थः benevolent, profitable to others

(xi) भवति *bhavati* = is, becomes

When the resolve of the *yogī* becomes firm towards truth, not towards the result, the deeds of that *yogī* become benevolent to others.

Comments : The yogi who is resolved to truth, is benevolent.

2.37 अस्तेयप्रतिष्ठायां सर्वरत्नोपस्थानम् ।

asteyapratiṣṭhāyam sarvaratnopasthānam

(asteya-pratiṣṭhāyam sarva-ratno-pasthānam)

(o) अस्तेय-प्रतिष्ठायाम् *asteya-pratiṣṭhāyam* =

(i) यदा योगिनः *yadā yoginaḥ* = when the yogī's

(ii) अस्तेयं प्रति *asteyam prati* = towards non-theft

(iii) दृढा भावना भवति *dṛḍha bhāvanā bhavati* = becomes firm conviction

(iv) तदा तं योगिनम् *tadā yoginam* = then to that yogī

(o) सर्व-रत्न-उपस्थानम् *sarva-ratno-pasthānam* =

(v) सर्वाणि *sarvāṇi* = all

(vi) रत्नानि *ratnāni* = श्रेष्ठवस्तुनि, परमलाभाः supreme gains

(vi) यदृच्छया एव *yadṛćchayā eva* = स्वयं एव by themselves

(viii) प्राप्नुवन्ति *prāpnuvanti* = come.

When the *yogī's* conviction towards non-theft becomes firm, then to that *yogī* all supreme gains come by themselves.

Comments : The yogi who does not steal, all supreme gains come to him.

ब्रह्मचर्यम् ।

brahmacharyam

37. Celibacy

2.38 ब्रह्मचर्यप्रतिष्ठायां वीर्यलाभः ।

brahmaćaryapratiṣṭhāyam vīryalābhaḥ

(brahmaćarya-pratiṣṭhāyam vīrya-lābhaḥ)

(o) ब्रह्मचर्य-प्रतिष्ठायाम् *brahmaćarya-pratiṣṭhāyam* =

(i) यदा योगिनः *yadā yoginaḥ* = when the yogī's

(ii) ब्रह्मचर्यं प्रति *brahmaćaryam prati* = towards celibacy

(iii) दृढा भावना भवति *dṛḍha bhāvanā bhavati* = becomes firm conviction

(iv) तदा सः योगी *tadā saḥ yogī* = then that yogī

(v) वीर्यलाभः *vīryalābhaḥ* = सामर्थ्य-लाभं प्राप्नोति attains power

When the *yogī's* conviction towards celibacy becomes firm, then that *yogī* attains power.

Comments : The abstinent yogi is powerful.

अपरिग्रहः ।

aparigrahaḥ

38. Abstinance

2.39 अपरिग्रहस्थैर्ये जन्मकथन्तासंबोधः ।

aparigrahasthairyam janmakathantāsambudhaḥ

(aparigraha-sthairyam janma-kathantāsambudhaḥ)

(o) अपरिग्रह-स्थैर्ये *aparigraha-sthairyam* =

(i) यदा योगिनः *yadā yoginaḥ* = when the yogī's

(ii) अपरिग्रहं प्रति *aparigraham prati* = त्यागम् प्रति असेवनम् प्रति towards non-possession

(iii) दृढा भावना भवति *dṛḍha bhāvanā bhavati* = becomes firm conviction

(iv) तदा *tadā* = then

(v) सः योगी *saḥ yogī* = that yogī

(vi) जन्म-कथन्ता-संबोधः *janma-kathantāsambudhaḥ* = knows his births

(vii) तस्य पूर्वजन्मानि जानाति *tasya pūrva-janmāni jānāti* = knows his previous lives

📖 **When the *yogī's* conviction towards non-possession becomes firm, then that *yogī* knows his previous lives.**

✍ Comments : The non-hoarding yogi knows his previous lives.

शौचः ।

śaucaḥ

39. Purity

2.40 शौचात्स्वाङ्गजुगुप्सा परैरसंसर्गः ।

śaucātsvāṅgajugupsā parairsaṁsargaḥ

(śaucāt-svāṅga-jugupsā parair-saṁsargaḥ)

(i) शौचात् *śaucāt* = शौचस्य, पावित्र्यस्य, धार्मिकत्वस्य, शुद्धेः of purity

(ii) पालनात् *pālanāt* = from the observance

(iii) स्वाङ्ग-जुगुप्सा *svāṅga-jugupsā* = निज-देहे वैराग्यं प्राप्नोति develops non-attachment in his body

(iv) तथा *tathā* = and

(v) सः योगी *saḥ yogī* = that yogī

(vi) अपरैः सह *aparai sah* = from others

(vii) अ-संसर्गः *saṁsargaḥ* = असंसर्गं, एकाकी, असम्मर्दम् lonelyness

(viii) इच्छति *icchati* = desires

📖 **From the <u>observance</u> of purity, the *yogī* develops non-attachment in his body and he desires loneliness from others.**

✍ Comments : Purity gives the nature of a sage i.e. a *muni* (Gita 2:56).

2.41 सत्त्वशुद्धिसौमनस्यएकाग्र्येन्द्रियजयाआत्मदर्शनयोग्यत्वानि ।

sattvaśuddhisaumanasyaekāgryendriyajayātmadarśanayogyatvāni

(sattva-śuddhi-saumanasya-ekāgrya-indriya-jaya-ātma-darśana-yogyatvāni)

(i) च *cha* = and

(o) सत्त्व-शुद्धि-सौमनस्य-एकाग्र्य-इन्द्रिय-जय-आत्म-दर्शन-योग्यत्वानि *sattva-śuddhi-saumanasya-ekāgryendriya-jayātma-darśana-yogyatvāni* =

(ii) सत्त्वं *sattvam* = सद्भावः righteousness

(iii) शुद्धिः *śuddhi* = पावित्र्यम् purity

(iv) सौमनस्य-एकाग्र्यं *saumanasya-ekāgram* = चेतसः एकता one-pointedness

(v) इन्द्रिय-जयः *indriya-jayaḥ* = इन्द्रियाणां निग्रहः self-control

(vi) आत्म-दर्शनं *ātma-darśanam* = स्व-परिक्षण-बुद्धिः self-examination

(vii) योग्यत्वं *yogyatvam* = आत्मसाक्षात्कारस्य योग्यता worthyess for self-revelation

(viii) इति अन्तःशुद्धेः *iti antaḥ-shuddheḥ* = of internal sanctity

(ix) पञ्च फलानि *pañca phalāni* = the five results

(x) लक्षणानि वा *lakṣaṇāni vā* = or signs

(xi) सन्ति *santi* = are

📖 **And, (i) <u>righteousness</u>, (ii) <u>purity</u>, (iii) <u>one-pointedness</u>, (iv) <u>self-control</u>, (v)** and worthyness for self-examination and self-revelation - are the five results or signs of internal sanctity.

सन्तोषः ।

santoṣaḥ

40. Contentment

2.42 सन्तोषादनुत्तमसुखलाभः ।

santoṣādanuttamasukhalābhaḥ *(santoṣād-anuttama-sukha-lābhaḥ)*

(i) सन्तोषात् *santoṣāt* = वितृष्णायाः समाधानात् from contentment

(o) अनुत्तम-सुख-लाभः *anuttama-sukha-lābhaḥ* =

(ii) अनुत्तमछ *anuttama:* = सर्वोत्तमः, परमः supreme

(iii) सुख-लाभः *sukha-lābhaḥ* = शान्तेः प्राप्तिः attainment of peace

(iv) भवति *bhavati* = is, becomes

📖 **From contentment comes attainment of supreme peace.**

तपः ।

tapaḥ

41. Austerity

2.43 कायेन्द्रियसिद्धिरशुद्धिक्षयात्तपसः ।

kāyendriyasiddhiśuddhikṣayāttapasaḥ

(kāye-ndriya-siddhir-śuddhi-kṣayāt-tapasaḥ)

(i) तपसः *tapasaḥ* = from austerity

(ii) प्रभावात् *prabhāvat* = from the influence, effect

(iii) च *cha* = and

(iv) अशुद्धि-क्षयात् *aśuddhi-kṣayāt* = अशुद्धेः नाशात् from the removal of impurity

(v) च *cha* = and

(o) काया-इन्द्रिय-सिद्धिः *kāyā-ndriya-siddhiḥ* =

(vi) कायायाः *kāyāyaḥ* = कायस्य, देहस्य of the body

(vii) इन्द्रियाणां च *indriyāṇām cha* = and of the organs

(viii) सिद्धिः *siddhiḥ* = साफल्यम्, कृतकार्यता competence, success

(ix) भवति *bhavati* = is, becomes

📖 **From the effect of (i) austerity and (ii) removal of impurity - becomes <u>competence</u> of the body and of the organs.**

✍ Comments : Austerity gives competence.

स्वाध्यायः ।

svādhyāyaḥ

42. Study of Scriptures

2.44 स्वाध्यायादिष्टदेवतासम्प्रयोगः ।

svādhyāyādiṣṭadevatāsamprayogaḥ

(svādhyāyād-iṣṭa-devatāsam-prayogaḥ)

(i) स्वाध्यायात् *svādhyāyāt* = वेद-शास्त्राभ्यासात् from the study of scriptures

(o) इष्ट-देवता-सम्प्रयोगः *iṣṭa-devatāsam-prayogaḥ* =

(ii) इच्छितायाः *icćhitāyāḥ* = वाञ्छितायाः, अभिलषितायाः of the desired

(iii) देवतायाः *devatāyāḥ* = दैवतस्य, देवस्य of the deity

(iv) साक्षात्कारः *sākṣātkāraḥ* = revelation

(v) भवति *bhavati* = is, becomes, occurs

📖 **From the study of scriptures occurs revelation of the desired deity.**

ईश्वरप्रणिधानम् ।

īśvarapraṇidhānam

43. Faith in God

2.45 समाधिसिद्धिरीश्वरप्रणिधानात् ।

samādhisiddhirīśvaraparṇidhānāt

(samādhi-siddhir-īśvara-parṇidhānāt)

(o) ईश्वर-प्रणिधानात् *īśvara-parṇidhānāt* =

(i) ईश्वरं प्रति *īśvaram prati* = भगवत: प्रति, भगवन्तं प्रति towards god

(ii) प्रणिधानात् *parṇidhānāt* = श्रद्धाया:, निष्ठाया:, भक्ते: from the faith

(o) समाधि-सिद्धि: *samādhi-siddhiḥ* =

(iii) समाधे: *samādheḥ* = of samādhiḥ, of meditation

(iv) सिद्धि: *siddhiḥ* = साफल्यं, पूर्णत्वं, कृतकार्यता success

(v) भवति *bhavati* = is, becomes, occurs

📖 **From the faith towards God occurs <u>success</u> in *samādhiḥ* (meditation).**

✍ Comments : Faith gives success is meditation.

आसमन् ।

āsanam

44. Steady State

2.46 स्थिरसुखमासनम् ।

sthirasukhamāsanam *(sthira-sukham-āsanam)*

(i) स्थिर-सुखम् *sthira-sukham* = steady with ease.

(ii) सुखेन *sukhena* = अव्यथया with ease

(iii) प्राप्ता *prāptā* = attained

(iv) स्थिरा स्थिति: *sthirā sthitiḥ* = steady state, stable position

(v) 'आसनम्' 'āsanam'

(vi) इति उच्यते *iti uchyate* = is known as, is called as

📖 **The steady state attained with ease is called as *'āsanam.'***

✍ Comments : *Asana* is the steady state of yoga.

2.47 प्रयत्नशैथिल्यानन्तसमापत्तिभ्याम् ।

prayatnaśaithilyānantasamāpattibhyām

(prayatna-śaithilyānanta-samāpattibhyām)

(o) प्रयत्न-शैथिल्य-अनन्त-समापत्तिभ्याम् *prayatna-śaithilyānanta-samāpattibhyām* =

(i) तत् आसनं *tat āsanam* = that āsana

(ii) प्रयत्न-शैथिल्यात् *prayatna-śaithilyāt* = अ-घोर-प्रयत्नात् without severe struggle

(iii) अनन्तस्य च *anantasya cha* = परमेश्वरस्य and with god

(iv) समापत्त्या: *samāpattyāḥ* = सम्पादनात्, संयोगात् from union with

(v) च *cha* = and

(vi) भवति *bhavati* = is, becomes, occurs

📖 **That *āsanam* occurs without severe struggle and from the union with God.**

✍ Comments : Asana occurs easily by union with God. That steady state is called *samadhi*.

द्वन्द्वातीतता ।

dvandvātītatā

45. Indifference to Duality

2.48 ततो द्वन्द्वानभिघातः ।

tato dvandvãnabhighātaḥ *(tato dvandvā-nabhighātaḥ)*

(i) ततः *tataḥ* = तदनु, तस्य आसनस्य सिद्धेः पश्चात् after successful attainment of the āsanam for samādhiḥ

(o) द्वन्द्व-अनभिघातः *dvandva-nabhighātaḥ* =

(ii) द्वन्द्वस्य *dvandvasya* = द्वन्द्वभावस्य of the thoughts of duality

(iii) आघातः *āghātaḥ* = आक्रमणम्, प्रक्षेपः influence, affect

(iv) न भवति *na bhavati* = does not occur

📖 **After successful attainment of the *āsanam* for *samādhiḥ*, one does not get affected by the thoughts of duality (influence of the thoughts of duality does not occur).**

✍ Comments : With successful *samadhi*, thoughts do not conflict.

प्राणायामः ।

prāṇāyāmaḥ

46. Breath Control

2.49 तस्मिन्सति श्वासप्रश्वासयोर्गतिविच्छेदः प्राणायामः ।

tasminsati śvāsapraśvāsayorgativicchedaḥ prāṇāyāmaḥ

(tasmin-sati śvāsa-pra-śvāsayor-gati-vicchedaḥ prāṇāyāmaḥ)

(i) तस्मिन् सति *tasmin-sati* = तस्य आसनस्य सिद्धौ in the success of the āsanam of the siddhiḥ

(ii) श्वास-प्रश्वासयोः = श्वासस्य = of the inbreath

(iii) प्रश्वासस्य च *pra-śvāsayoḥ cha* = उच्छ्वासस्य, निःश्वासस्य and of outbreath

(o) गति-विच्छेदः *gati-vicchedaḥ* =

(iv) गतेः *gateḥ* = चलनस्य, सरणस्य, वेगस्य of the rate of

(v) विच्छेदः *vicchedaḥ* = वियोगः, लवनम् control

(vi) 'प्राणायामः' = 'prāṇāyāmaḥ'

(vii) इति उच्यते *iti uchyate* = is known as, is called as

📖 **In the success of the *āsanam* of the *siddhiḥ*, the control of the rate of the in-breath and of out-breath, is called as *'prāṇāyāmaḥ.'***

✍ Comments : *Pranayama* is the control breathing. It is required or the success of *asana*.

2.50 बाह्याभ्यन्तरस्तम्भवृत्तिर्देशकालसंख्याभिः परिदृष्टो दीर्घसूक्ष्मः ।

bāhyābhyantarastambhavṛttirdeśakālasaṅkhyābhiḥ paridṛṣṭo dīrghasūkṣmaḥ;

(bāhyābhyantara-stambha-vṛttir-deśa-kāla-saṅkhyābhiḥ pari-dṛṣṭo dīrgha-sūkṣmaḥ)

(o) बाह्य-आभ्यन्तर-स्तम्भ-वृत्तिः *bāhyābhyantara-stambha-vṛttiḥ* =

(ii) बाह्यवृत्तिः *bāhya-vṛttiḥ* = उच्छ्वासस्य अवस्था the rate of outbreath

(iii) आभ्यन्तरवृत्तिः *abhyantara-vṛttiḥ* = श्वासस्य अवस्था the rate of inbreath

(iv) स्तम्भवृत्तिः च *stambha-vṛttiḥ cha* = श्वास-उच्छ्वासयोः स्तम्भनस्य अवस्था and the rate of holding the breath

(v) इति त्रिविधाः *iti tridhāḥ* = these three ways of

(vi) प्राणायामाः = *praṇāyāmas*

(vii) भवन्ति *bhavanti* = are

(o) देश–काल–संख्याभि: *deśa-kāla-saṅkhyābhiḥ* =

(viii) स्थानस्य *sthānasya* = of the place

(ix) समयस्य *samayasya* = of the time

(x) संख्याया: *saṅkhyāyāḥ* = क्रमस्य, अभीक्ष्णताया:, पौन्यस्य of the frequency

(xi) अनुसारेण *anusāreṇa* = according to

(xii) परिदृष्टि: *pari-dṛṣṭiḥ* = सम्यक् निरीक्षणं कृत्वा by properly observing

(o) दीर्घ–सूक्ष्म: *dīrgha-sūkṣmaḥ* =

(xiii) दीर्घ: *dīrgha-sūkṣmaḥ* = long

(xiv) वा लघु: *vā laghuḥ* = or short

(xv) प्राणायाम: *prāṇāyamaḥ* = the prāṇāyama, the breathing

(xvi) भवति *bhavati* = is, becomes, occurs

📖 **The (i) rate of out-breath, the (ii) rate of in-breath and the (iii) rate of holding the breath are three ways of *praṇāyāmas.* By properly observing the rate, the *prāṇāyamaḥ* becomes long or short according to the place, the time and the frequency;**

✍ Comments : The fourth type (iv) is given in the next sutra.

2.51 बाह्याभ्यन्तरविषयाक्षेपी चतुर्थ: ।

bāhyābhyantaraviṣayākṣepī ćaturthaḥ

(bāhyā-bhyantara-viṣayākṣepī ćturthaḥ)

(o) बाह्य–आभ्यन्तरे–विषय–आक्षेपी *bāhyā-bhyantara-viṣayākṣepī* =

(i) बाह्यानां *bāhyānām* = of the external

(ii) अभ्यन्तराणां च *abhyantarābhyām cha* = and of the internal

(iii) विषयानां त्यागात् *viṣayānām tyāhāt* = by keeping away the thoughts

(iv) 'चतुर्थः' *'ćaturthaḥ'* = the fourth

(v) इति नाम्नः *iti nāmnaḥ* = called

(vi) प्रणायामः *prāṇāyamaḥ* = prāṇāyām, breathing

(vii) स्वयम् एव भवति *syayam eva bhavati* = occurs automatically

📖 **by (v) keeping away the external and the internal thoughts, the *prāṇāyamaḥ* that occurs automatically is called *'ćaturthaḥ,'* (the fourth) *prāṇāyamaḥ*.**

✍ Comments : The influence of this fourth type of *pranayama* is given in the next sutra.

2.52 ततः क्षीयते प्रकाशावरणम् ।

tataḥ kṣīyate prakāṣāvaraṇam (*tataḥ kṣīyate prakāṣāvaraṇam*)

(i) ततः *tataḥ* = तस्य 'चतुर्थस्य' प्राणायामस्य अभ्यासात् from the accomplishment of the fourth prāṇayāmaḥ

(ii) प्रकाश–आवरणम् *prakāṣa-āvaraṇam* = प्रकाशस्य, ज्ञानं आच्छादयमानम् masking the light of knowledgs

(iii) आवरणं *āvaraṇam* = आच्छादनं, पिधानम् the covering

(iv) क्षीयते *kṣīyate* = क्षीणः भवति, निःसरति gets dissolved, is removed

📖 **From the accomplishment of the fourth *prāṇayāmaḥ,* the covering that is masking the light of knowledge, gets dissolved.**

2.53 धारणासु च योग्यता मनसः ।

dharaṇāsu ća yogyatā manasaḥ (*dharaṇāsu ća yogyatā manasaḥ*)

(i) च *cha* = एवं च similarly

(ii) धारणासु *dharaṇāsu* = ध्येये, चित्तस्य स्थिर-बन्धने in the stability of thoughts

(iii) मनसः *manasaḥ* = of mind

(iv) योग्यता *yogyatā* = क्षमता, सामर्थ्यम्, युक्तता, ओचित्यम् vigor, conditioning

(v) भवति *bhavati* = is, becomes, occurs

📖 **Similarly, from the stability of thoughts occurs conditioning of mind.**

✍ Comments : The steady state conditions the mind.

प्रत्याहारः ।

pratyāhāraḥ

47. Conditioning

2.54 स्वविषयसम्प्रयोगे चित्तस्वरूपानुकार इवेन्द्रियाणां प्रत्याहारः ।

svaviṣayasamprayoge ćittasvarūpānukāra ivendriyāṇām pratyāhāraḥ

(sva-viṣaya-samprayoge ćitta-svarūpā-nukāra ive-ndriyāṇām pratyāhāraḥ)

(i) स्व-विषय-सम्प्रयोगे *sva-viṣaya-samprayoge* = स्वेषां विषयाणां क्षये by keeping away the internal and external thoughts

(ii) इन्द्रियाणां स्वरूपं *ive-ndriyāṇām svarūpam* = the nature of sense organs

(iii) स्वप्रकृतेः *sva-pṛkṛteḥ samānam* = चित्त-स्वरूपानुकारः इव analogous to one's own original inborn nature

(iv) भवनम् *bhavanam* = becoming of

(v) 'प्रत्याहारः' *pratyāhāraḥ*

(vi) इति उच्यते *iti uchyate* = is known as, is called as

📖 **Making of the nature of sense organs analogous to one's own original inborn**

nature, by keeping away the internal and external thoughts, is called as *'pratyāhāraḥ* (conditioning).'

✍ Comments : *Pratyahara* is conditioning of the mind. Mind is conditioned in meditation by keeping external thoughts away and keeping sense organs according to one's own inborn nature. For five sense organs, see verse 2.20 above.

2.55 ततः परमा वश्यतेन्द्रियाणाम् ।

tataḥ paramā vaśyatendryāṇām *(tataḥ paramā vaśyate-ndryāṇām)*

(i) ततः *tataḥ* = तेन प्रत्याहारेण = with that pratyāhāraḥ

(ii) इन्द्रियाणां *indriyāṇām* = of the organs

(iii) परमा *paramā* = पूर्णः = total

(iv) वश्यता *vaśyatā* = निग्रहः, संयमः control

(v) भवति *bhavati* = becomes, occurs

📖 **With that *pratyāhāraḥ,* occurs total control of the organs.**

✍ Comments : *Pratyahara* gives self control.

3. विभूतिपादः ।

vibhūtipādaḥ

धारणा ।

dhāraṇā

48. Steady Abstraction

3.1 देशबन्धश्चित्तस्य धारणा ।

deśabandhaścittasya dhāraṇā

(deśa-bandha-ścittasya dhāraṇā)

(i) देश-बन्धः *deśa-bandhaḥ* = stabilizing in place, keeping collected

(ii) चित्तस्य *cittasya* = of mind

(iii) धारणा *dhāraṇā* = 'dhāraṇā,' steady abstraction of mind

(iv) इति उच्यते *iti uchyate* = is known as, is called as

🕮 **Stabilizing of mind in place is called as *'dhāraṇā'* (steady abstraction of mind)**

ध्यानम् ।

dhyānam

49. Concentration

3.2 तत्र प्रत्ययैकतानता ध्यानम् ।

tatra pratyaiktānatā dhyānam *(tatra pratyai-ktānatā dhyānam)*

(i) तत्र *tatra* = देहस्य बहि: वा अभ्यन्तरे वा outside or inside the body =

(ii) यत्र चित्तं स्तब्धं तिष्ठति तत्र एव *yatra chittam stabdham tiṣṭhati tarta eva* = wherever the mind stays in steady abstraction

(o) प्रत्यय-एकतानता *pratya-ektānatā* =

(iii) प्रत्ययस्य *pratyasya* = वृत्ते: of the absorption

(iv) एकतानता *ektānatā* = एकाग्रता, एक-सूत्रता the one-pointedness

(v) 'ध्यानम्' *'dhyānam,'* = meditation

(vi) इति उच्यते *iti uchyate* = is known as, is called as

Outside or inside the body, wherever the mind stays in steady abstraction, the one-pointedness of the absorption is called as *'dhyānam'* (concentration).

Comments : One pointed meditation on the aim is *dhyanam.*

समाधि: ।

samādhiḥ

50. Meditation

3.3 तदेवार्थमात्रनिर्भासं स्वरूपशून्यत्वमिव समाधि: ।

tadevārthamātranirbhāsam svarūpaśūnyatvamiva samādhiḥ

(tat-evā-rtha-mātra-nirbhāsam svarūpa-śūnyatvam-iva samādhiḥ)

(o) अर्थमात्र-निर्भासम् *artha-mātra-nirbhāsam* =

(i) यदा ध्याने *yadā dhyāne* = while concentrating when

(ii) ध्येयस्य *dhyeyasya* = of the aim

(iii) प्रतीति: *pratītiḥ* = बोध: the perception

iv) एव अवशिष्यते *eva avaṣisyate* = only remains

v) तथा *tahtā* = and

o) स्वरूप-शून्यत्वम्-इव *svarūpa-śūnyatvam-iva* =

vi) चित्तस्य *chittasya* = of mind

vii) निज-स्वरूपं *nija-svarūpam* = the own nature

viii) शून्यत्वम् इव *śūnyatvam* = अविद्यमानम् इव like emptiness, like vacuum

ix) भवति *bhavati* = is, becomes, occurs

x) तदा *tadā* = then

xi) सा स्थितिः *sa sthitiḥ* = that state

xiii) 'समाधिः' *'samādhiḥ'* = meditation

xiv) इति उच्यते *iti uchyate* = is called as

📖 **While concentrating, when only the perception of the aim remains and the own nature of mind becomes like vacuum, then that state is called as *'samādhiḥ'* (meditation).**

✍ Comments : The *dhyanam*, in which one becomes oblivious own nature, is *samadhi*.

संयमः ।

saṁyamaḥ

51. Restraint

3.4 त्रयमेकत्रम् संयमः ।

trayamekatram saṁyamaḥ *(trayam-ekatram saṁyamaḥ)*

(i) त्रयम् *trayam* = the three, namely :

(ii) धारणा *dhāraṇā* = the steady abstraction

(iii) ध्यानं *dhyānam* = concentration

(iv) समाधिः च *samādhi cha* = and meditation

(v) यदा *yadā* = when

(vi) एकत्रं *ekatram* = एक–ध्येये in one goal

(vii) वर्तन्ते *vartante* = exist

(viii) तदा *tadā* = then

(ix) सः ध्येयत्रयः *saḥ dhyetrayaḥ* = that trio of goals

(x) 'संयमः' *'saṁyamaḥ'* = restraint

(xi) इति उच्यते *iti uchyate* = is known as, is called as

📖 **When the steady (i) abstraction, (ii) concentration and (iii) meditation exist in one goal, then that trio of goals is called as *'saṁyamaḥ'* (restraint).**

✍ Comments : The steady trio of abstraction, concentration and meditation is *samyam*.

प्रज्ञालोकः ।

prajñālokaḥ

52. Light of Cognition

3.5 तज्जयात्प्रज्ञालोकः ।

tajjayātprajñālokaḥ *(taj-jayāt-prajñā-lokaḥ)*

(i) तत् *tat* = तस्य संयमस्य of that restraint

(ii) जयात् *jayāt* = वशात् with the attainment, control

(o) प्रज्ञा–आलोकाः *prajñā-lokaḥ* =

(ii) प्रज्ञायाः *prajñāyāḥ* = ज्ञानस्य of understanding, enlightened state

(iv) आलोकः *ālokaḥ* = प्रकाशः, विद्यमानता, आविर्भावः existence, manifestatiom

(v) वर्तते *vartate* = occurs

📖 **With the attainment of that restraint, manifestation of enlightened state occurs.**

✍ Comments : The trio of *samyam* gives enlightened state to the *yogi.*

3.6 तस्य भूमिषु विनियोगः ।

tasya bhūmiṣu viniyogaḥ *(tasya bhūmiṣu viniyogaḥ)*

(i) तस्य *tasya* = तस्य संयमस्य of that restraint

(ii) भूमिषु *bhūmiṣu* = विषयेषु, अर्थेषु, स्थानेषु in the objects

(iii) विनियोगः *viniyogaḥ* = स्थूल-सूक्ष्म-क्रमेण in a proper order from material to subtle objects

(iv) उपयोगः *upyogaḥ* = प्रयोगः, संयम-प्रयोगः the application

(v) करणीयः *karaṇīyaḥ* = should be done

📖 **The application of that restraint should be done in a proper order from material to subtle objects.**

✍ Comments : The aim of meditation should be gradual from material to subtle objects.

अन्तरङ्गम् ।

antarangam

53. Interior

3.7 त्रयमन्तरङ्गं पूर्वेभ्यः ।

trayamantaraṅgam pūrvebhyaḥ *(trayam-antaraṅgam pūrvebhyaḥ)*

(i) पूर्वेभ्यः *pūrvebhyaḥ* = उपरोक्तेभ्य from the above mentioned

(ii) अष्ट अङ्गेभ्यः *aṣṭ-angebhyaḥ* = यम-नियम-आसन-प्राणायम-प्रत्याहार-धारणा-ध्यान-समाधिः इति eight components namely : (1) Self control, (2) observance, (3) posture, (4) breath control, (5) withholding, (6) focus on aim (7) concentration and (8) meditation (see 2.29↑)

(iii) त्रयम् *trayam* = एतत् साधना त्रयं, धारणा, ध्यानम्, समाधिः this trio of sādhanā namely : (1) focus on aim (2) concentration and (3) meditation

(iv) योगसिद्धौ *yogasiddhau* = in the yogasiddhi, in the success of yoga

(v) 'अन्तरङ्गम्' *'antarangam,'* = the central core

(vi) अस्ति *asti* = is

📖 **The above mentioned eightfold path of components namely (i) Self control, (ii) observance, (iii) posture, (iv) breath control, (v) withholding, (vi) focus on aim (vii) concentration and (viii) meditation, this forms the trio of *sādhanā* namely (i) focus on aim (ii) concentration and (iii) meditation - is the *'antarangam,'* (the central core) in the *'yogasiddhi'* (the success of yoga) or the *'sādhanā.'***

✍ Comments : The eightfold *antarangam* is the central core of success of the yoga.

बहिरङ्गम् ।

bahirangam

54. Exterior

3.8 तदपि बहिरङ्गम् निर्बिजस्य ।

tadapi bahirangam nirbījasya *(tad-api bahir-angam nir-bījasya)*

(i) तत् *tat* = उपरोक्तं *uparoktam* = the above mentioned

(ii) साधना-त्रयम् *sādhanā-trayam* = trio of sādhanā

(iii) अपि *api* = also

(iv) निर्बीजस्य *nirbījasya* = निर्बीज-समाधेः of the nirbīja samādhiḥ, meditation without any source of influence see 1.51

(v) बहिरङ्गम् *bahir-angam* = बाह्य–अङ्गम् the exterior component

(vi) अस्ति *asti* = is

📖 **The above mentioned octave of *sādhanā* is the exterior component of the *nirbīja samādhiḥ* (the meditation without any source of influence).**

✍ Comments : *Sadhana* is the exterior component of nir-beeja-damadhi.

3.9 व्युत्थाननिरोधसंस्कारयोरभिभवप्रादुर्भावौ निरोधक्षणचित्तान्वयो निरोधपरिणामः ।

vyutthānanirodhasam̐skārayorabhibhavaprādurbhāvau nirodhakṣaṇaćittānvayo nirodhapariṇāmaḥ

(vyutthāna-nirodha-sam̐skārayor-abhibhava-prādurbhāvau nirodha-kṣaṇa-ćittānvayo nirodha-pariṇāmaḥ)

(o) व्युत्थान–निरोध–संस्कारयोः *vyutthāna-nirodha-sam̐skārayoḥ* =

(i) संस्कारस्य *sam̐skārasya* = of the sam̐skāraḥ = of the impression on the mind

(ii) व्युत्थानं *vyutthānam* = वृत्तेः अवरोध hinderence of impression on mind

(iii) निरोधः *nirodhaḥ* = वृत्तेः लयः melting, disappearance, dissolution of impression on mind

(iv) अवस्थायोः *avasthāyoḥ* = in the two states

(o) अभिभव–प्रादुर्भावौ *abhibhava-prādurbhāvau* =

(v) संस्कारस्य *sam̐skārasya* = of the impression on the mind

(vi) अभिभवः *abhibhavaḥ* = आधिक्यं, प्राबल्यं, सर्गः upsurge

(vii) प्रादुर्भाव *prādurbhāva* = विकाश, विकास, अवतरणं appearance

(viii) अवस्थायोः *avasthāyoh* = of the two states

(o) निरोध–क्षण–चित्त–अन्वयः *nirodha-kṣaṇa-ćitta-anvayaḥ* =

(ix) निरोधस्य *nirodha* = of hinderence

(x) क्षणे *kṣaṇe* = समये, काले at the time of

(xi) चित्तस्य *ćittasya* = मनसः, चेतसः of mind

(xii) निरोधः *nirodhaḥ* = निग्रहः, संयमः control

(xiii) संस्कारानुसारेण *saṁskārānusāreṇ* = संस्कारवत् according to impressions

(xiv) भवनम् *bhavanam* = becoming according to impressions on mind

(xv) 'निरोधपरिणामः' *'nirodha pariṇāmaḥ,'* = consequence of restraint

(xvi) इति उच्यते *iti uchyate* = is called as

📖 **In the two states namely : (i) hindrance and (ii) dissolution of the impression on the mind, and in the two states namely : (i) appearance and (ii) upsurge of the impression on the mind, the control of mind according to the impressions is called as the '*nirodha pariṇāmaḥ*' (consequence of restraint).**

✍ Comments : The control of mind according to the impressions on the mind is *nirodha-parinama.*

3.10 तस्य प्रशान्तवाहिता संस्कारात् ।

tasya praśāntavāhitā saṁskārāt *(tasya praśānta-vāhitā saṁskārāt)*

(i) संस्कारात् *saṁskārāt* = तस्य संस्कारस्य प्रभावात्, तस्मात् मानस्यां शिक्ष्याम् from that impression on mind

(ii) तस्य *tasya* = तस्य चित्तस्य, मनसः, चेतसः of mind

(iii) प्रशान्ता *praśānta* = क्षोभहीना, निश्चला, स्तिमिता, निष्कम्पा, उद्वेगशून्या tranquil

(iv) वाहिता *vāhitā* = प्रवाहिता, प्रवृत्ता, प्रेरिता, सञ्चारिता, ऊढा flowing

(v) स्थितिः *sthitiḥ* = the state

(vi) 'प्रशान्तवाहिता' *'praśāntavāhitā'* = calmly streaming

(vii) इति उच्यते *iti uchyate* = is known as, is called as

📖 **From that diminished impression on mind, the tranquil flowing state of mind is called as *'praśāntavāhitā'* (calmly streaming state).**

✍ Comments : The streaming of impressions from diminished state to tranquil flowing state is *prashanta-vahita.*

3.11 सर्वार्थतैकाग्रतयोः क्षयोदयौ चित्तस्य समाधिपरिणामः ।

sarvārthataikāgratayoḥ kṣayodayau ćittasya samādhipariṇāmaḥ

(sarvārtha-taikāgratayoḥ kṣayo-dayau ćittasya samādhi-pariṇāmaḥ)

(o) सर्वार्थता-एकाग्रतयोः *sarvārtha-taikāgratayoḥ* =

(i) सर्वेषु *sarveṣu* = in all

(ii) अर्थेषु *sarvārtheṣu* = विषयेषु in the matters

(iii) चित्तवृत्तेः *ćittavṛtteḥ* = एकाग्रस्य चिन्तनस्य अवस्थायाः of the state of one-pointedness of mind

(o) क्षयः-उदयः *kṣaya-udayaḥ* =

(iv) क्षयः *kṣayḥ* = अपचयः, ह्रासः the decline, diminution, decay, wane

(v) च एके अर्थे (विषये) *cha eka arthe* = and in any one matter

(vi) चित्तवृत्तेः *ćittavṛtteḥ* = चिन्तनस्य उदयः, उद्गमः, आविर्भावः rise, increase of the state of one-pointedness of mind

(vii) 'समाधि-परिणामः' *'samādhi-pariṇāmaḥ,'* = product or consequence of meditation

(viii) इति उच्यते *iti uchyate* = is known as, is called as

📖 **The diminution of all matters in the state of one-pointedness of mind with the increase in the state of <u>one-pointedness of mind in any one matter</u> is called as *'samādhi-pariṇāmaḥ'* (consequence of meditation).**

✍ Comments : The diminution of all matters to one-pointed state and increase of this one-pointedness on only one matter is *samadhi-parinama.*

एकाग्रता ।

ekāgratā

55. One-pointedness

3.12 ततः पुनः शान्तोदितौ तुल्यप्रत्ययौ चित्तस्यैकाग्रतापरिणामः ।

tataḥ punaḥ śāntoditau tulyapratyayau ćittasyaikāgratāpariṇāmaḥ

(tataḥ punaḥ śānto-ditau tulya-pratyayau ćittasyai-kāgratāpariṇāmaḥ)

(i) ततः *tataḥ* = तदनु, तत् पश्चात् thereafter

(ii) पुनः *punaḥ* = again

(iii) यदा *yadā* = when

(iv) शान्त–उदितौ *śānta-uditau* = शान्तवृत्तिः, क्षोभहीना, निश्चला, स्तिमिता, निष्कम्पा, उद्वेगशून्या tranquility, calmness

(v) उदिता वृत्तिः च *uditā vṛttiḥ cha* = क्षुब्धा, चञ्चला वृत्तिः and unrest

(vi) तुल्य–प्रत्ययौ *tulya-pratyayau* = यदा समानौ भवतः when both come to an equilibrium

(vii) तदा *tadā* = then

(viii) चित्तस्य स्थितिः *ćittasya avasthā* = तस्य चेतसः अवस्था that state of mind

(ix) 'एकाग्रता–परिणामः' *'ekāgratā-pariṇāmaḥ,'* = consequence of one-pointedness

(x) इति उच्यते *iti uchyate* = is known as, is called as

📖 **Thereafter, again when tranquility and unrest both come to an equilibrium, then that state of mind is called as *'ekāgratā-pariṇāmaḥ'* (consequence of one-pointedness).**

✍ Comments : The state where tranquility and unrest of mind come to an equilibrium, is *ekagtata-parinama.*

3.13 एतेन भूतेन्द्रियेषु धर्मलक्षणावस्थापरिणामा व्याख्याता ।

etena bhūtendriyeṣu dharmalakṣaṇāvasthāpariṇāmā vyākhyātā

(etena bhūte-ndriyeṣu dharma-lakṣaṇā-vasthā-pariṇāmā vyākhyātā)

(i) एतेन *etena* = उपरोक्तेन परिणामेन with the consequences mentioned above. see 3:9, 10, 11 and 12 above.

(ii) भूतेन्द्रियेषु *bhūtendriyeṣu* = पञ्चभूतेषु च एकादश इन्द्रियेषु च in the five basic-elements and eleven organs namely five work organs, five sense organs and mind

(o) धर्म–लक्षण–अवस्था–परिणामाः *dharma-lakṣaṇā-vasthā-pariṇāmāḥ* =

(iii) धर्म–परिणामः *dharma-pariṇāmaḥ* = एकस्य गुणस्य क्षयः अन्यस्य च गुणस्य उदयः diminution of one matter in the state of one-pointedness of mind

(iv) लक्षण–परिणामः *lakṣaṇā-vasthā-pariṇāmāḥ* = एकस्य गुणस्य प्रभावस्य क्षयः अन्यस्य च गुणस्य प्रभावस्य उदयः and increase of ther matter in the state of one-pointedness of mind

(v) अवस्था–परिणामः च *avasthā-pariṇāmāḥ cha* = गुणप्रभावस्य एकस्याः स्थितेः क्षयः अन्यस्थितेः उदयः and, increase of the influence of one of the three attributes in the in the state of one-pointedness of mind

(vi) व्याख्याताः *vyākhyātāḥ* = उक्ताः, उपरोक्ताः described

(vii) सन्ति *santi* = are

📖 **The above consequences in the state of one-pointedness of mind are thus described : (i) the diminution of one matter in the state of one-pointedness of mind; (ii) and increase of the matter in the state of one-pointedness of mind; (iii) and increase of the influence of one of the three *guṇas* (attributes) - (in the five basic-elements and eleven organs, namely five work organs, five sense organs and mind).**

धर्मी ।

dharmī

56. Righteous

3.14 शान्तोदिताव्यपदेश्यधर्मानुपाति धर्मी ।

śāntoditāvyapadeśyadharmānupāti dharmī

(śānto-ditāvyapadeśya-dharmānupāti dharmī)

(0) शान्त-उदित-अव्यपदेश्य *śānta-udita-avyapadeśya* =

(i) शान्तः *śāntaḥ* = अतीतः, गतः past

(ii) उदितः *uditaḥ* = वर्तमानः, आविर्भूतः, प्रकाशितः, प्रकटितः active, present

(iv) अव्यपदेश्यं च *avyapadeśyam cha* = अविष्यः, आगामी and future

(o) धर्म-अनुपाति *dharma-anupati* =

(v) अनुपाती *anupāti* = attitude

(vi) अस्ति *asti* = is, that is present in

(vii) सः धर्मः *sah dharmaḥ* = सः गुणः, लक्षणम्, शक्तिः, स्वभावः the rectitude, virtue

(viii) 'धर्मी' *'dharmī,'* = righteous

(ix) इति उच्यते *iti uchyate* = is known as, is called as

🕮 **The virtue that is present in the past, present and future attitudes, is called as *'dharmī'* (righteous).**

✍ Comments : Virtue in the attitude is *dharmi.*

हेतुः परिणामः च ।

hetuḥ pariṇāmaḥ ća

57. Reason and Result

3.15 क्रमान्यत्वं परिणामान्यत्वे हेतुः ।

kramānyatvam pariṇāmānyatvam hetuḥ

(kramā-nyatvam pariṇamā-nyatvam hetuḥ)

(i) परिणाम-अन्यत्वे = परिणामस्य, विक्रियायाः, निष्पत्तेः of the consequence

(ii) अन्यत्वे *anyatve* = भिन्नतायाम् in the difference

(iii) क्रम-अन्यत्वम् *krama-anyatvam* = तेषां क्रमस्य, अनुक्रमस्य, पारम्पर्यस्य, विरचनस्य in the result of their sequence or order

(iv) अन्यत्वं *anyatvam* = भिन्नता, पृथक्त्वम् for the different result

(v) हेतुः *heuḥ* = कारणम् the reason

(vi) अस्ति *asti* = is

📖 **The reason for the difference in results of the consequence is their sequence.**

✍ Comments : Their sequence is the reason for the difference in the results.

3.16 परिणामत्रयसंयमादतीतानागतज्ञानम् ।

pariṇāmatrayasam̐yamādatītānāgatajñānam

(pariṇāma-traya-sam̐yamād-atītān-āgata-jñānam)

(i) परिणाम-त्रय-संयमात् *pariṇāma-traya-sam̐yamād* =

(ii) उपरोक्तस्य *uparoktasya* = of the three consequences mentioned above see 3.13

(iii) परिणामत्रयस्य *pariṇāma-trayasya* = धर्म-परिणामस्य च लक्षण-परिणामस्य च अवस्था-परिणामस्य च the three consequences, namely :

(1) the diminution of one matter in the state of one-pointedness of mind;

(2) and increase of the matter in the state of one-pointedness of mind;

(3) and increase of the influence of one of the three guṇas (attribute) in the state of one-pointedness of mind.

(iv) संयमात् *sam̐yamāt* = निग्रहात्, नियन्त्रणात्, मर्यादापालनात् with the control over

(o) अतीत-अनागत-ज्ञानम् *atīta-anāgata-jñānam* =

(v) अतीतस्य *atītasya* = भूतस्य, गत-कालस्य of the past

(vi) अनागतस्य च *anāgatasya cha* = भविष्यस्य, आगामी-कालस्य and future matters

(vii) ज्ञानं *jñānam* = knowledge

(viii) भवति *bhavati* = becomes, occurs, happens

📖 **With the control over the three consequences mentioned above, namely (i) the diminution of one matter in the state of one-pointedness of mind; (ii) and increase of the matter in the state of one-pointedness of mind; (iii) and increase of the influence of one of the three *guṇas* (attribute) in the state of one-pointedness of mind, knowledge of the past and future matters comes.**

✍ Comments : Knowledge of the past and future comes with the meditation on the above mentioned three consequences.

रुतज्ञानम् ।

rutajñānam

58. Perception of Speech

3.17 शब्दार्थप्रत्ययानामितरेतराध्यासात्सङ्करस्तत्प्रविभागसंयमात्सर्व-भूतरुतज्ञानम् ।

śabdārthapratyānāmitaretarādhyāsātsaṅkarastatpravibhāgasaṁyamāt-sarvabhūtarutajñānam

(śabdārtha-pratyānām-itaretarā-dhyāsāt-saṅkaras-tat-pravibhāga-saṁyamāt-sarva-bhūta-ruta-jñānam)

(i) शब्दार्थ-प्रत्ययानाम् *śabdārtha-pratyānām* = 'शब्द-अर्थ-ज्ञान' इति प्रत्ययत्रयस्य of the three distinct aspects, namely the name, form and understanding

(ii) इतरेतर-अध्यासात् *itaretarā-dhyāsāt* = एकस्मिन् अन्यस्य अध्यासात्, आसनात्, प्रतीतेः the study of intertwined relationship

(iii) सङ्करः *saṅkaraḥ* = संमेलनं, मेलनम्, संमिश्रणम् intermixture

v) भवति *bhavati* = becomes, occurs, happens

o) तत्-प्रविभाग-संयमात् *tat-pravibhāga-saṁyamāt* =

v) तस्मिन् *tasmin* = in that

vi) विभागे *vibhāge* = क्षेत्रे, विषये in that field, in that area, in that subject

vii) संयमनं कृत्वा *(saṁyamanam kṛtvā* = having meditated up on

o) सर्व-भूत-रुत-ज्ञानम् *sarva-bhūta-ruta-jñānam* =

viii) सर्वेषां भूतानां *sarveshām bhūtānām* = of all beings

ix) वाण्याः *vāṇyāḥ* = भाषायाः, वाचः, गिरः of the language

x) ज्ञानं *jnānam* = the knowledge

xi) भवति *bhavati* = is, becomes, occurs, happens

Having meditated up on the field of study of intertwined relationship of the intermixture of three distinct aspects, namely the (i) name, (ii) form and (iii) understanding, comes the knowledge of the language of all beings.

Comments : Knowledge of the language of all beings comes from the meditation on their name, form and understanding.

पुनर्जन्म ।

punarjanma

59. Reincarnation, rebirth

3.18 संस्कारसाक्षात्कारणात्पूर्वजातिज्ञानम् ।

saṁskārasākṣātkāraṇatpūrvajātijñānam

(saṁskāra-sākṣāt-kāraṇat-pūrva-jāti-jñānam)

(o) संस्कार-साक्षात्-कारणात् *saṁskāra-sākṣāt-kāraṇat* =

(i) जन्मजन्मनां *janma-janmanām* = of the previous births

(ii) संगृहितान् *saṅgṛhitān* = the accumulated

(iii) संस्कारान् *saṁskārān* = impressions on mind

(iv) साक्षात् *sākṣāt* = प्रत्यक्षान्, गोचरान् कृत्वा having realized, visualized, seen, brought infront

(o) पूर्व-जाति-ज्ञानम् *pūrva-jāti-jñānam* =

(v) पूर्वजन्मनां *pūrva-janmanām* = of previous births, previous lives

(vi) ज्ञानम् *jñānam* = knowledge

(viii) भवति *bhavati* = becomes, occurs, happens

📖 **Having realized the accumulated impressions of previous births on mind, comes knowledge of previous births.**

✍ Comments : Knowledge of previous births comes from the meditation on accumulated impressions of previous births.

परचित्तज्ञानम् ।

parachittajñānam

60. Intuition

3.19 प्रत्ययस्य परचित्तज्ञानम् ।

pratyasya parachittajñānam *(pratyasya para-chitta-jñānam)*

(i) प्रत्ययस्य *pratyasya* = अन्यस्य चित्तस्य of other's mind

(ii) साक्षात्कारं कृत्वा *sākshātkāram kṛtvā* = having perceivedrealized, with the perception of

(iii) पर-चित्त-ज्ञानम् *para-chitta* = अन्यस्य चित्तस्य of other's thoughts

(iv) ज्ञानं *jñānam* = knowledge

(v) भवति *bhavati* = becomes, occurs, happens

📖 **With the perception of other's mind comes the knowledge of other's**

thoughts.

✍ Comments : Knowledge of other's thoughts comes from the meditation on perception of other's mind.

3.20 न च तत्सालम्बनं तस्याविषयीभूतत्वात् ।

na ća tatsālambanam tasyāviṣayaībhūtatvāt

(na ća tat-sā-lambanam tasyā-viṣayaī-bhūtatvāt)

(i) च *cha* = and = परन्तु however

(ii) तत् *tat* = तत् ज्ञानम् that knowledge

(iii) न स–आलम्बनम् *na sa ālambanam* = न आलम्बनेन, न चित्तस्य ध्येयेन not of the actual content

(iv) सहितम् *sahitam* = is only of the form of other's thought

(v) न विद्यते *na vidyate* = is not

(vi) यतः *yataḥ* = because

(vii) तस्य अविषयी–भूतत्वात् *tasyā-viṣayaī-bhūtatvāt* = अन्यस्य भूतस्य चिन्तनस्य विषयः the subject of other's thinking

(viii) अन्यः *anyaḥ* = भिन्नः, अगम्यः external matter even to his mind

(ix) भवति *bhavati* = is, becomes, occurs, happens to be

📖 **However, that knowledge is only of the form of other's thought but not of its actual content, because the subject of other's thinking is external matter even to his mind.**

✍ Comments : The content of other's thoughts being external to his mind, knowledge of his thought comes but its actual content.

अन्तर्धानम् ।

antardhānam

61. Becoming Invisible

3.21 कायरूपसंयमात्तद्ग्राह्यशक्तिस्तम्भे चक्षुःप्रकाशासम्प्रयोगेऽन्तर्धानम् ।

kāyarūpasam̃yamãttadgrāhyaśaktistambhe

ćakṣuḥprakāśāsamprayoge'ntardhānam

(kāya-rūpa-sam̃yamãt-tat-grāhya-śakti-stambhe

ćakṣuḥ-prakāśāsamprayoge-'ntar-dhānam)

(o) काय-रूप-संयमात् *kāya-rūpa-sam̃yamãt* =

(i) कायस्य *kāyasya* = शरीरस्य of the body

(ii) रूपस्य *rūpasya* = स्वरूपस्य, स्वभावस्य of the true nature

(iii) संयमात् *sam̃yamãt* = संयमनं कृत्वा, निग्रहं कृत्वा having meditated up on

(o) तत्-ग्राह्य-शक्तिः स्तम्भे *tat-grāhya-śakti-stambhe* =

(iv) अन्येषां *anyeshām* = of others

(vi) तं योगिनं *tam yoginam* = to that yogī, that yogī

(vii) ग्रहणं कर्तुं *grahaṇam kartum* = to perceive, seeing

(viii) सामर्थ्यं *sāmarthyam* = ability

(ix) स्तम्भे *stambhe* = स्तब्धं भवति, अवरुद्धं भवति becomes suspended

(o) चक्षु-प्रकाश-असम्प्रयोगे *ćakṣuḥ-prakāśāsamprayoge* =

(x) अन्यस्य चक्षुणोः *anyasya chakshuṇoḥ* = अन्यस्य नेत्रयोः of other's eyes

(xi) प्रकाशस्य *prakāśasya* = दर्शनशक्तेः of power of vision

(xii) तेन सह असम्प्रयोगे *tena saha a-samprayoge* = तस्य सम्बन्धस्य अभावे with the disjunction of the connection

(xiii) अन्तर्धानम् *antardhānam* = Invisible

(xiv) सः योगी *saḥ yogī* = that yogī

(xv) अन्येषां अन्तर्धानः *anyeshām antardhānaḥ* = अदृश्यः, अदर्शनीयः, अलक्ष्यः, अप्रेक्षणीयः, परोक्षः, दर्शनातीतः, अरूपः invisible or unperceivable

(xvi) भवति *bhavati* = is, becomes, occurs, happens

📖 **Having meditated up on his body, the ability of other people to perceive that *yogī,* becomes suspended. With the disjunction of the connection of power of vision of other's eyes, that *yogī* becomes invisible or unperceivable.**

✍ Comments : The knowledge to become invisible comes from the meditation on one's own body.

मृत्युज्ञानम् ।

mṛtyujñānam

62. Knowledge of Death

3.22 सोपक्रमं निरूपक्रमं च कर्म तत्संयमादपरान्तज्ञानमरिष्टेभ्यो वा ।

sopakramam nirūpakramam ća tatsaṁyamādaparāntajñānamariṣṭebhyo vā

(so-pakramam nirūpa-kramam ća tat-saṁyamād-aparānta-jñānam-ariṣṭebhyo vā)

(i) स–उपक्रमम् *sa-upakramam* = उपक्रमेण, फलारम्भेण, उपायज्ञानपूर्वकारम्भेण सहितः the *karmas* which have started rendering their fruit

(ii) कर्म = कर्मणि = the karmas which

(iii) निरूपक्रमम् च *nirūpa-kramam ća* = उपक्रम विरहितः च have not yet started rendering their fruit and

(iv) वा *vā* = अथवा = and, or

(v) तत्–संयमात् *tat-saṁyamāt* = तस्य संयमनं कृत्वा, तन्निगृहित्य by meditating up on

(vi) अरिष्टेभ्यः *ariṣṭebhyaḥ* = अशुभेभ्यः, अपशकुनेभ्यः from misfortunes

(vii) चिह्नेभ्यः *chinhebhyaḥ* = लक्षणेभ्यः from signs

(viii) अ-परान्त-ज्ञानम् *aparānta* = अपरान्त, मृत्योः of death

(ix) ज्ञानं *jñānam* = knowledge

(x) भवति *bhavati* = becomes, occurs, happens

🕮 **By meditating up on the *karmas* which have started rendering their fruit and the *karmas* which have not yet started rendering their fruit, comes the knowledge of the signs of misfortunes and of one's death.**

✍ Comments : The knowledge to foresee the fortunes and misfortunes comes from meditation on *karmas* that have and that have not yielded fruit.

हस्तिबलम् ।

hastibalam

63. Strength like an Elephant

3.23 मैत्र्यादिषु बलानि ।

maitryādiṣu balāni *(maitry-ādiṣu balāni)*

(o) मैत्री-आदिषु *maitrī ādiṣu* =

(i) मैत्री *maitrī* = मित्रत्वम्, सौहृद्यम्, सखित्वम्, बन्धुता, स्नेहः, प्रीतिः by meditating up on friendship

(ii) करुणा *karuṇā* = दया, अनुकम्पा, कृपा compassion

(iii) मुदिता *muditā* = आनन्दः, प्रसन्नता happiness

(iv) आदिषु *ādiṣu* = = ...etc.

(v) बलानि *balāni* = प्रभावाः, सामर्थ्यम्, क्षमता, शक्तिः corresponding strengths

(vi) आगच्छन्ति *āgacchanti* = come

🕮 **By meditating up on friendship, compassion, happiness ...etc. corresponding strengths come.**

✍ Comments : The knowledge of earning corresponding strength comes from meditating on friendship, compassion, happiness, etc.

3.24 बलेषु हस्तिबलादीनि ।

baleṣu hastibalādīni *(baleṣu hasti-balādīni)*

(i) बलेषु *baleṣu* = प्रभावेषु एकाग्रं कृत्वा by meditating up on strengths

(ii) हस्तिबल-आदीनि *hasti-bala-ādīni* = हस्ति-व्याघ्र-भीम-सदृशाः like those of elephant, tiger, Bhima ...etc.

(iii) प्रभावाः *prabhāvāḥ* = powers

(iv) योगी *ypgī* = the yogī

(v) प्राप्नोति *prāpnoti* = attains

📖 **By meditating up on strengths, the *yogī* attains powers like those of elephant, tiger, Bhima ...etc.**

✍ Comments : The knowledge to earn power like an elephant comes from meditation on those strengths.

दूरवस्तुज्ञानम् ।

dūravastujñānam

64. Knowledge of Remote Objects

3.25 प्रवृत्त्यालोकन्यासात्सूक्ष्मव्यवहितविप्रकृष्टज्ञानम् ।

pravṛttyālokanyāsātsūkṣmavyavahitaviprakṛṣṭajñānam

(pravṛttyāloka-nyāsāt-sūkṣma-vyavahita-viprakṛṣṭa-jñānam)

(o) प्रवृत्ति-आलोक-न्यासात् *pravṛtti-āloka-nyāsāt* =

(i) एतादृश्या: *etādṛshyāḥ* = by meditating up on such objects as :

(ii) ज्योतिष्मत्या: *jotishmatyāḥ* = प्रभाविन्या: enlightened

(iii) वृत्या: *vṛtyāḥ* = states (see 1.36 and 3.5 above)

(iv) प्रखरस्य आलोकस्य *ptakharasya ālokasya* = clear vision

(v) न्यासात् *nyāsāt* = किरणपतनात्, प्रतिक्षेपात्, परावर्तनात् being unable to be seen

(o) सूक्ष्म-व्यवहित-विप्रकृष्ट-ज्ञानम् *sūkṣma-vyavahita-viprakṛṣṭa-jñānam* =

(vi) सूक्ष्माणां वस्तूनां *sūkṣmāṇām vastūnām* = of the subtle things

(vii) दूरस्थानां स्थितानां *dūrasthānām sthitānām* = located at a far distance

(viii) देशानां *deshānām* = भूभागानाम्, स्थलानाम्, क्षेत्राणाम्, स्थानानाम् of places

(ix) विषयानां *vastūnām* = वस्तूनाम् of things

(x) ज्ञानं *jñānam* = knowledge

(xi) भवति *bhavati* = becomes, occurs, happens

📖 **By meditating up on his enlightened states, the *yogī* attains knowledge of places and things located at a far distance and which are unable to be seen directly.**

✍ Comments : The knowledge of minute and remote objects comes from meditation on own enlightened states.

भुवनज्ञानम् ।

bhuvanajñānam

65. Knowledge of Universe

3.26 भुवनज्ञानं सूर्ये संयमात् ।

bhuvanajñānam sūrye samyamāt *(bhuvana-jñānam sūrye samyamāt)*

(i) सूर्ये *sūrye* = विश्वमण्डलस्य चिन्तनं भूमित: सूर्यपर्यन्तं of the planetary system from the earth to the sun

(ii) यदा *yadā* = when

(iii) योगी करोति *yogī karoti* = the yogī does

(iv) तदा *tadā* = then

(v) संयमात् *saṁyamāt* = तस्मात् संयमात्, अन्तर्ध्यानात्, समाधेः from that meditation

(vi) सः योगी *saḥ yogī* = that yogī

(o) भुवन-ज्ञानम् *bhuvana-jñānam* =

(vii) भुवनस्य *bhuvanasya* = भू-मण्डलस्य, चतुर्दश भुवन-मण्डलस्य of the fourteen worlds

(viii) ज्ञानं *jñānam* = understanding

(ix) प्राप्नोति *prāpnoti* = attains

📖 **When the *yogī* meditates up on the planetary system from the earth to the sun, then from that meditation that *yogī* attains understanding of the fourteen worlds.**

✍ Comments : The knowledge of fourteen worlds comes from meditation on the planetary system from earth to the Sun.

3.27 चन्द्रे ताराव्यूहज्ञानम् ।

ćandre tārāvyūhajñānam *(ćandre tārā-vyūha-jñānam)*

(i) चन्द्रे *ćandre* = विश्वमण्डलस्य चिन्तनं भूमितः चन्द्रपर्यन्तं of the planetary system from the earth to the moon

(ii) यदा *yadā* = when

(iii) योगी करोति *yogī karoti* = the yogī does

(iv) तदा *tadā* = then

(v) संयमात् *saṁyamāt* = तस्मात् संयमात्, अन्तर्ध्यानात्, समाधेः from that meditation

(vi) सः योगी *saḥ yogī* = that yogī

(vii) तारा-व्यूह-ज्ञानम् *tārā-vyūha-jñānam* = तारागण-मण्डलस्य, द्यु-मण्डलस्य of the earth and its planets

(viii) ज्ञानं *jñānam* = understanding

(ix) प्राप्नोति *prāpnoti* = attains

📖 **When the *yogī* meditates up on the planetary system from the earth to the moon, then from that meditation that *yogī* attains understanding of the earth and its planets.**

✍ Comments : The knowledge of the earth and its planets comes from the meditation on planetary system from earth to the Moon.

3.28 ध्रुवे तद्गतिज्ञानम् ।

dhruve tadgatijñānam *(dhruve tad-gati-jñānam)*

(i) ध्रुवे *dhruve* = विश्वमण्डलस्य ध्यानं भूमितः ध्रुव-उड्डु-पर्यन्तं of the planetary system from the earth to the Northern star

(ii) यदा *yadā* = when

(iii) योगी करोति *yogī karoti* = the yogī does

(iv) तदा *tadā* = then

(v) संयमात् *saṁyamāt* = तस्मात् संयमात्, अन्तर्ध्यानात्, समाधेः from that meditation

(vi) सः योगी *saḥ yogī* = that yogī

(vii) तद् *tad* = उड्डु-मण्डलस्य = of the planetary system

(viiii) गतिः *gatiḥ* = व्रजनस्य अवस्थायाः of the motion and state

(ix) ज्ञानं *jñānam* = understanding

(x) प्राप्नोति *prāpnoti* = attains

📖 **When the *yogī* meditates up on the planetary system from the earth to the Northern star, then from that meditation that *yogī* attains understanding of the motion and state of the planetary system.**

✍ Comments : The knowledge of motion and states of the planetary system comes from the meditation on planetary system from the earth to the Northern star.

3.29 नाभिचक्रे कायव्यूहज्ञानम् ।

nābhićakre kāyavyūhajñānam *(nābhi-ćakre kāya-vyūha-jñānam)*

(i) नाभिचक्रे *nābhi-ćakre* = तुन्दकूपौ on the belly button where all the nerves are tied together *kaṇṭha-kūpe*

(ii) संयमनं कृत्वा *saṁyamanam kṛtvā* = by meditation up on

(iii) योगी *yohī* = the yogī

(o) काया–व्यूह–ज्ञानम् *kāya-vyūha-jñānam* =

(iv) कायस्य *kāyasya* = कायाया:, शरीरस्य of the body

(v) व्यूहस्य *vyūhasya* = सर्वासां नाडीनां स्नायूनां अस्थीनां गात्राणां अवयवानां च of all the nerves, muscles, veins, arteries, bones and organs

(vi) सम्यक् *samyak* = proper

(vii) ज्ञानं *jñānam* = understanding

(viii) प्राप्नोति *prāpnoti* = attains

📖 **by meditation up on the belly button, where all the nerves are tied together, the *yogī* attains proper understanding of all the nerves, muscles, veins, arteries, bones and organs.**

✍ Comments : Knowledge of all body organs comes from the meditation on the belly button.

क्षुत्पिपासानिवृत्तिः ।

kṣutpipāsānivṛttiḥ

66. Hunger and Thirst Control

3.30 कण्ठकूपे क्षुत्पिपासानिवृत्तिः ।

kaṇṭhakūpe kṣutpipāsanivṛttiḥ *(kaṇṭha-kūpe kṣut-pipāsa-nivṛttiḥ)*

(i) कण्ठकूपे *kaṇṭha-kūpe* = गलस्य रन्ध्रे at the opening of the throat

(ii) संयमनं कृत्वा *samyamanam kṛtvā* = by meditating up on

(iii) योगिनः *yoginaḥ* = of the yogī

(o) क्षुत्-पिपासा-निवृत्तिः *kṣut-pipāsa-nivṛttiḥ* =

(iv) क्षुधायाः *kṣudhāyāḥ* = जिघत्सायाः, बुभुक्षायाः of hunger

(v) पिपासायाः च *pipāsāyāḥ cha* = तृष्णायाः, उदन्यायाः, तृषायाः च and of thirst

(vi) निवृत्तिः *nivṛttiḥ* = निवारणम्, विलोपः cessation

(vii) भवति *bhavati* = becomes, occurs, happens

📖 **By meditating at the opening of the throat, cessation of hunger thirst of the *yogī* occurs.**

✍ Comments : The knowledge to conquer hunger and thirst comes from the meditation on the opening of the throat.

कुण्डलीनिविद्या ।

kuṇḍalanividyā

67. Knowledge of Energy Centers

3.31 कूर्मनाड्यां स्थैर्यम् ।

kūrmanāḍyām sthairyam *(kūrma-nāḍyām sthairyam)*

(i) कूर्मनाड्याम् *kūrma-nāḍyām* = वक्षस्थलस्य कूर्मनाड्यां on the turtle shaped nerve below the chest

(ii) संयमनं कृत्वा *samyamanam kṛtvā* = by meditating up on

(iii) योगी y*ogī* = the yogī

(iv) स्थैर्यम् *sthairyam* = स्थिरतां steady state of the body and mind

(v) प्राप्नोति *prāpnoti* = attains

📖 **By meditating up on the turtle shaped nerve below the chest the *yogī* attains steady state of the body and mind.**

✍ Comments : The knowledge to rest the body and mind in steady state comes from the meditation on the turtle shaped nerve below the chest.

3.32 मूर्धज्योतिषि सिद्धदर्शनम् ।

mūrdhjyotiṣi siddhadarśanam *(mūrdh-jyotiṣi siddha-darśanam)*

(i) मूर्ध-ज्योतिषि *mūrdh-jyotiṣi* = कपोलस्य ब्रह्य-रन्ध्रस्य ज्योते: at the aperture in the crown of the head through which the atmā is supposed to escape on leaving the body

(ii) संयमनं कृत्वा *samyamanam kṛtvā* = by meditating up on

(iii) योगी y*ogī* = the yogī

(iv) सिद्ध-दर्शनम् *siddha-darśanam* = दिव्य-सिद्धानां दर्शनं, सक्षात्कारम् revelation of all the divine sages

(v) प्राप्नोति *prāpnoti* = attains

📖 **By meditating up on the aperture in the crown of the head through which the *ātmā* is supposed to escape on leaving the body, the *yogī* attains revelation of all the divine sages.**

✍ Comments : The knowledge all divine sages comes from the meditation on the aperture in the crown of the head.

सर्वज्ञानम् ।

sarvajñānam

68. Universal Knowledge

3.33 प्रातिभाद्वा सर्वम् ।

prātibhatdvā sarvam *(prātibhat-vā sarvam)*

(i) प्रातिभात् वा *prātibhat-vā* = प्रतिभ-ज्ञानात् and from the the meditation of the precursor of thinking

(i) योगी *yogī* = the yogī

(i) सर्वम् *sarvam* = सर्वज्ञानं *sarva-jñānam* = omniscience

(v) प्राप्नोति *prāpnoti* = attains

🕮 **From the meditation of the <u>precursor of thinking</u> the *yogī* attains omniscience.**

✍ Comments : Omniscience comes from the meditation on the precursor of thinking.

आत्मज्ञानम् ।

ātmajñānam

69. Self Realization

3.34 हृदये चित्तसंवित् ।

hṛdaye ćittasamvit *(hṛdaye ćitta-samvit)*

(i) हृदये *hṛdaye* = चित्ते, चेतसि, हृदि, आत्मनि on his own heart

(ii) संयमनं कृत्वा *samyamanam kṛtvā* = by meditating up on

(iii) योगी *yogī* = the yogī

(iv) चित्त-संवित् *ćitta-samvit* = चित्तस्य, आत्मनः, स्वस्य of himself

(v) सर्वज्ञानं *sarva-jñānam* = complete understanding

(vi) प्राप्नोति *prāpnoti* = attains

📖 **By meditating up on his own heart, the *yogī* attains complete understanding of himself.**

✍ Comments : The knowledge on oneself comes from meditation on own heart.

3.35 सत्त्वपुरुषयोरत्यन्तासङ्कीर्णयोः प्रत्ययाविशेषो भोगः परार्थात्स्वार्थसंयमात्पुरुषज्ञानम् ।

sattvapuruṣayoratyantāsaṅkīrṇayoḥ pratyāviśeṣo bhogaḥ parārthātsvārthasam̃yamātpuruṣajñānam

(sattva-puruṣayor-atyantā-saṅkīrṇayoḥ pratyāviśeṣo bhogaḥ parā-rthāt-svārtha-sam̃yamāt-puruṣa-jñānam)

(o) सत्त्व-पुरुषयोः *sattva-puruṣayoḥ* =

(i) सत्त्वस्य *sattvasya* = पंचभूतानां च त्रिगुणानां च, प्रकृतेः of the prakṛtiḥ i.e. of mahā-bhūtas (the five basic-elements) and the guṇas (the three-attributes)

(ii) पुरुषस्य च *puruṣasya* = आत्मनः च = and of the atmā

(o) अत्यन्त-सङ्कीर्णयोः *atyantā-saṅkīrṇayoḥ* =

(iii) अत्यन्तः *atyantaḥ* = अमितः, अतीव, भूरि, सुष्ठु intricately

(iv) असङ्कीर्णः *asaṅkīrṇaḥ* = मिश्रितः, अस्पष्टः, मिश्रः, सङ्करितः mixed

(o) प्रत्यय-अविशेषः *pratyāviśeṣaḥ* =

(v) अविशेषः *aviśeṣaḥ* = अभेद्यः, अपृथक्करणीयः the non-analyzable

(vi) प्रत्यय: *pratyaḥ* = प्रतीति:, ज्ञानम्, बोध: understanding

(vii) 'भोग:' *'bhogaḥ,'* = experience

(viii) इति उच्यते *iti uchyate* = is known as, is called as

(ix) परार्थात् *para-arthāt* = परस्य अर्थात्, पर हेतो: from the purpose of others

(x) भिन्न: य: स्वार्थ: अस्ति *bhinnaḥ yaḥ svārthaḥ asti* = स्व हेतु: that which is different from one's own purpose

(xi) तस्मात् संयमनात् *tasmāt samỹamanāt* = तस्मिन् संयमनं कृत्वा by meditating on that

(xii) पुरुष-ज्ञानम् *puruṣa-jñānam* = पुरुषस्य अभिन्नत्वस्य ज्ञानम् understanding of one's indifference with puruṣaḥ

(xiii) आयाति *āyāti* = comes

📖 **The non-analyzable understanding of (i) the intricately mixed *prakṛtiḥ* i.e. of *mahā-bhūtas* viz. five basic-elements and the *guṇas* viz. three-attributes and (ii) of the ātmā, is called as *'bhogaḥ'* (experience).**

On meditating on the purpose of others, which is different from one's own purpose, comes understanding of one's indifference with *puruṣaḥ*.[1]

✍ Comments : The knowledge of one's own difference from the *purusha* comes from the meditation on the difference between own purpose from other's purpose.

भुवनज्ञानम् ।

bhuvanajñānam

70. Knowledge of Universe

3.36 तत: प्रातिभश्रावणवेदनादर्शास्वादवार्ता जायन्ते ।

[1] For a very clear understanding on terms such as *Prakriti, purusha, atmā*, please see my publication *"Gita as She is in Krishna's Own Words"* Volume I, you will greatly benefit. See it on www.books-india.com

tataḥ prātibhaśrāvaṇavedanādarśāsvādavārtā jāyante

(tataḥ prātibha-śrāvaṇa-vedanādarśāsvāda-vārtā jāyante)

(i) ततः *tataḥ* = तस्मात् पुरुषज्ञानात् with such understanding of puruṣa

(o) प्रातिभ-श्रावण-वेदन-आदर्श-आस्वाद-वार्ता *prātibha-śrāvaṇa-vedanādarśāsvāda-vārtā* =

(ii) प्रातिभस्य *prātibhasya* = प्रतिभायाः, प्रज्ञायाः of actual perception of subtle, hidden or distant things of past, present and future

(iii) श्रावणस्य *śrāvaṇasya* = श्रावणिकस्य, श्राव्य being able to hear inaudible sounds

(iv) वेदनस्य *vedanasya* = वेदनायाः, स्पर्शस्य being able to feel spiritual touch

(v) आदर्शस्य *ādarśasya* = दर्शनस्य, अवलोकनस्य, ईक्षणस्य being able to see divine forms

(vi) आस्वादस्य *āsvādasya* = रसनस्य, स्वादनस्य, वासस्य, गन्धस्य being able to taste things from thought only

(vii) वार्ताः *vārtā* = being able to smell abstract things

(viii) ज्ञानानि जायन्ते *jñāni jāyante* = one attains knowledge of

📖 **With that understanding of the *puruṣa,* one attains success in (i) being able for actual perception of subtle, hidden or distant things of past, present and future, (ii) being able to hear inaudible sounds (iii) being able to feel spiritual touch, (iv) being able to see divine forms (v) being able to taste things from thought only and (vi) being able to smell abstract things.**

✍ Comments : The knowledge of above mentioned six things comes from the meditation on the *purusha.*

सिद्धिः ।

siddhiḥ

71. Success[2]

---

[2] Many translators and tutors have misunderstood this word and translated as "perfection." When one attains *siddhi* in a *yoga*, it does not mean he attained perfection, and there is no room for improvement. *Siddhi* means one has

3.37 ते समाधावुपसर्गाः व्युत्थाने सिद्धयः ।

te samādhāvupasargāḥ vyutthāne siddhayaḥ

(te samādhā-vupasargāḥ vyutthāne siddhayaḥ)

(i) ते *te* = उपरोक्ता: षट्-सिद्धय: the above mentioned are six successes (see 3.36)

(ii) समाधौ *samādhau* = समाधि-सिद्धौ in meditation

(iii) उपसर्गा: सन्ति *vupasargāḥ santi* = बाधा:, उपद्रवा:, विघ्नानि there are imperfections in them

(iv) परन्तु *parantu* = but

(v) व्युत्थाने *vyutthāne* = व्युत्थितौ in paradox

(vi) ता: सिद्धय: सन्ति *tāḥ aiddhayaḥ santi* = they are the successes

📖 **The above mentioned are six successes in meditation, but there are imperfections in them, therefore, they are the successes in paradox.**

✍ Comments : Above mentioned are the six kinds of apparent success in meditation.

परदेहप्रवेशः ।

paradehapraveśaḥ

72. Entering in Other's Body

3.38 बन्धकारणशैथिल्यात्प्रचारसंवेदनाच्च चित्तस्य परशरीरावेशः ।

bandhakāraṇaśaithilyātpracārasaṃvedanāc ca

---

successfully attained that yoga to a desired degree. According to the Upanishadic philosophy, **nothing is perfect**, other than *brahma.* Something that has no room for absolutey any improvement, is perfect. Thus, Patañjali says, "there are hindrances." In this *sūtra*, the six *siddhis* are not six perfections but success that have imperfectiopns or hindrances.

ćittasya paraśarīrāveśaḥ

(bandha-kāraṇa-śaithilyāt-praćāra-saṁvedanāć ća ćittasya para-śarīrāveśaḥ)

(i) बन्ध–कारण *bandha-kāraṇa* = बन्धनैः कारणात् because of the tendency of karma's to form attachment

(ii) शैथिल्यात् *śaithilyāt* = शिथिलतायाः, दीर्घसूत्रतायाः, श्लघतायाः, व्यापेक्षात् the ātmā is bound the body

(iii) प्रचार–संवेदनात् तु *praćāra-saṁvedanāt tu* = आत्मनः but with meditation on ātmā

(iv) गतेः *gateḥ* = व्रजनस्य, गमनस्य, आवागमनस्य, अयनस्य, यानस्य, सरणस्य going out and coming in

(v) संवेदनात् *saṁvedana* = अनुभवात्, ज्ञानात्, बोधात् from the experience

(vi) चित्तस्य *ćittasya* = मनसः, चेतसः by mind

(o) पर–शरीर–आवेशः *para-śarīrāveśaḥ* =

(vii) पर *para* = अन्य, अपर = other's

(viii) शरीर *śarīra* = देहम्, कायाम्, तनुम् in the body

(ix) आवेशः *āveśaḥ* = गमनम्, प्रवेशः, निवेशः entering

(x) योगी कर्तुं शक्यते *yogī kartum shakyate* = the yogī can achieve

📖 **Because of the tendency of *karmas* to form attachment, the *ātmā* is bound with the body, but with meditation on *ātmā* and thus from the experience of going out and coming in, the *yogī* can achieve entering in other's body, by mind.**

✍ Comments : The knowledge to enter one's body comes from the meditation on *atma.*

3.39 उदानजयाज्जलपङ्ककण्टकादिष्वसङ्गुत्क्रान्तिश्च ।

udānajayājjalapaṅkakaṇṭakādiṣvasaṅgutkrāntiśća

(udāna-jayāj-jala-paṅka-kaṇṭakā-diṣva-saṅg-utkrāntiś ća)

(o) उदान–जयात् *udāna-jayāt* =

(i) उदानस्य *udānasya* = कण्ठस्य वायोः, हृदयतः तालु–पर्यन्तं चारिणः वायोः the breath that flows between heart and palate

(ii) जयात् *jayāt* = निग्रहात्, संयमात् by meditating on

(o) जल-पङ्क-कण्टक-आदिषु *jala-panka-kaṇṭakā-diṣu* =

(iii) जलेषु *jaleṣu* = अंभःसु, वारिषु, अप्सु in water

(iv) पङ्केषु *pankeṣu* = कर्दमेषु, जम्बालेषु in mud

(v) कण्टकेषु च *kaṇṭakeṣu cha* = शल्येषु, विघ्नेषु, शूलेषु and in thorns

(o) असङ्गः *asangaḥ* =

(vi) शरीरस्य सङ्गः *śarīrasya sangaḥ na bhavati* = संस्पर्शः, स्पर्शः, संसर्गः न भवति do not sink

(vii) परम् *param* = परन्तु but

(viii) उत्क्रान्तिः *utkrāntiḥ* = उर्ध्व-गतिः the yogī attains shukla-mārga when he dies

📖 **By meditating on the breath that flows between the heart and the palate, the *yogī* does not sink in water and mud (if he walks over them) and he attains death in *shukla-mārga* when he dies.**

✍ Comments : Knowledge of walking on water comes from the meditation on the breath that flows between the heart and the palate.

3.40 समानजयाज्ज्वलनम् ।

samānajayāj jvalanam *(samāna-jayāj jvalanam)*

(i) समान-जयात् *samāna-jayāt* = समान, नाभेः वायोः, हृदयतः नाभि-पर्यन्तं चारिणः वायोः, पाचक-वायोः the breath that flows between heart and belly-button

(ii) संयमनात् *samāna-jayāt* = निग्रहात् by meditating on

(iii) ज्वलनम् भवति *jvalanam bhavati* = योगिनः शरीरं ज्वलनं, दीप्तिमन्तम्, उज्ज्वलम्, भासुरम्, भास्वरम् भवति the body of the yogī becomes radiant

📖 **By meditating on the breath (*prāṇa*) that flows between the heart and the**

belly-button (through the blood stream), the body of the *yogī* becomes radiant.

✍ Comments : The knowledge to become radiant comes from the meditation on the breath that flows between the heart and the belly-button.

दिव्यश्रवणशक्तिः ।

divyaśravaṇaśaktiḥ

73. Microhearing

3.41 श्रोत्राकाशयोः सम्बन्धसंयमाद्दिव्यं श्रोत्रम् ।

śrotrākāśayoḥ sambandhasaṁyamāddivyam śrotram

(śrotrākā-śayoḥ sambandha-saṁyamāt divyam śrotram)

(o) श्रोत्र–आकाशयोः *śrotra- ākāśayoḥ* =

(i) *śrotrasya* = श्रोत्रस्य, कर्णस्य, शब्दस्य of sound

(ii) आकाशस्य *ākāśasya* = खेः, शब्दस्य of the sky and sound

(iii) सम्बन्ध–संयमात् *sambandha-saṁyamāt* = सम्बन्धस्य, संयोगस्य, संश्लेषस्य, सम्पर्कस्य निग्रहात् by meditating on the connection

(iv) योगिनः *yoginaḥ* = of the yogī

(v) श्रोत्रम् *śrotram* = श्रवणः, श्रुतिः, आकर्णनम्, निशमनम् hearing

(vi) दिव्यम् *divyam* = अलौकिकं, भास्वरम्, ऐश्वर्ययुक्तं, तीव्रम् super, supreme

(vii) भवति *bhavati* = becomes, occurs, happens

📖 **By meditating on the connection of the sky and sound, the *yogī* attains super hearing.**

✍ Comments : The knowledge of micro-hearing comes fro the meditation on the connection of the sky and sound.

आकाशगमनम् ।

ākāśagamanam

74. Aerial Travel

3.42 कायाकाशयोः सम्बन्धसंयमाल्लघुतूलसमापत्तेश्चाकाशगमनम् ।

kāyākāśayoḥ sambandhasaṁyamallaghutūlasamāpatteśchākāśagamanam

(kāyā-ākāśayoḥ sambandha-saṁyamal-laghu-tūla-samāpatteś-chākāśa-gamanam)

(o) काया–आकाशयोः *kāyā-ākāśayoḥ* =

(i) कायायाः *kāyāyāḥ* = देहस्य, शरीरस्य of the body

(ii) आकाशस्य च *ākāśasya cha* = खेः च and of the sky

(iii) सम्बन्ध–संयमात् *sambandha-saṁyamat* = सम्बन्धस्य, संयोगस्य, संश्लेषस्य, सम्पर्कस्य निग्रहात् by meditating on the connection between

(iv) योगिनः *yoginaḥ* = of the yogī

(v) शरीरम् *śarīram* = the body

(o) लघु–तूल–समापत्तेः *laghu-tūla-samāpatteḥ* =

(vi) तूल *tūla* = कर्पासः, पिचुलः, ऊर्णा, लोम cotton

(vii) इव *iva* = like

(viii) लघु *laghu* = लघुभारः, अल्पभारः light

(ix) भवति *bhavati* = is, becomes, occurs, happens

(x) एवं च *evam cha* = and

(xi) योगी *yogī* = the yogī

(o) आकाश–गमनम् *ākāśa-gamanam* =

(xii) आकाशे *ākāśe* = दिवि, अन्तरिक्षे, गगने, नभसि in the sky

(xiii) गमनं *gamanam* = चलनम्, भ्रमणम्, परिभ्रमणम्, पर्यटनम्, यात्रा, प्रवासः travel, fly

(xiv) कर्तुं शक्नोति *kartum śaknoti* = is able to do

📖 **By meditating on the connection between the body and the sky, the body of the *yogī* become light like cotton and the *yogī* is able to fly in the sky.**

✍ Comments : The knowledge of becoming light like cotton comes from the meditation on the connection between the body and the sky.

महाविदेहा

mahāvidehā

75. Aura

3.43 बहिरकल्पिता वृत्तिर्महाविदेहा ततः प्रकाशावरणक्षयः ।

bhirkalpitā vṛttirmahāvidehā tataḥ prakāśāvaraṇakṣayaḥ

(bhir-kalpitā vṛttir-mahāvidehā tataḥ prakāśāvaraṇa-kṣayaḥ)

(o) बहिः–अकल्पिता *bhiḥ-akalpitā* =

(i) बहिः *bhih* = शरीरस्य बहिः, बाह्यतः outside the body

(ii) अकल्पिता *akalpitā* = अकाल्पनिका, अकृत्रिमा, नैसर्गिका the natural

(iii) वृत्तिः *vṛttiḥ* = state

(iv) 'महाविदेहा' *mahāvidehā* = 'mahā-videhaḥ'

(v) इति उच्यते *iti uchyate* = is known as, is called as

(vi) ततः *tasmat* = तस्मात् therefore by meditating on that

(vii) महाविदेहा–वृत्तेः *mahā-videha vṛtteḥ = of the mahā-videha state*

(o) प्रकाश–आवरण–क्षयः *prakāśāvaraṇa-kṣayaḥ* =

(viii) प्रकाशस्य *prakāśasya* = ज्ञानस्य, बुद्धेः, विद्यायाः of thinking, mind

(ix) आवरणस्य *āvaraṇasya* = अज्ञान–रूपस्य आवरणस्य, भ्रमस्य the covering of ignorance

(x) क्षयः *kṣayaḥ* = नाशः, सारणम्, उच्छेदः, अपसारणम्, अज्ञान–खण्डनम् removal

(xi) भवति *bhavati* = becomes, occurs, happens

📖 **The natural state outside the body is called as *'mahā-videhaḥ.'* By meditating on that *mahā-videha* state, occurs removal of the covering of ignorance over thinking.**

✍ Comments : The knowledge of removing ignorance ace comes from the meditation on the natural state outside one's body.

पञ्चभूतप्रकृतिविजयः ।

pañćabhūtaprakṛtivijayaḥ

76. Conquering the Nature

3.44 स्थूलस्वरूपसूक्ष्मान्वयार्थवत्त्वसंयमाद्भूतजयः ।

sthūlasvarūpasūkṣmānvayārthavattvasaṁyamādbhūtajayaḥ

(sthūla-svarūpa-sūkṣmānvayār-thavattva-saṁyamāt bhūta-jayaḥ)

(o) स्थूल-स्वरूप-सूक्ष्म-अन्वय-अर्थवत्त्व-संयमात् *sthūla-svarūpa-sūkṣmānvayār-thavattva-saṁyamāt* =

(i) भूतानां *bhūtānām* = of the beings

(ii) स्थूला *sthūlā* = इन्द्रियगोचरा, शब्द-स्पर्श-रूप-रस-गन्धादि-पञ्च the five tangible ordres manely hearing, touch, form, taste and smell

(iii) स्वरूपा *svarūpā* = इन्द्रियागोचरा, स्वरूपमया, घनता-द्रवता-उष्णता-विरलता-विस्तीर्णता आदि पञ्च the five intangible orders namely solidity, fluidity, warmth, density and span

(iv) सूक्ष्मा *sūkṣmā* = तन्मात्रा च सूक्ष्म-भूतानि च the subtle elements

(v) अन्वयाः *anvayāḥ* = सत्-रजस्-तमसादि तिस्रः the three sat, rajas and tamas guṇas

(vi) अर्थवत्त्व *ārthavattva* = प्रयोजनता motive

(vii) इति पञ्च *iti pañcha* = these five

(viii) अवस्थानां *avasthānām* = of states

(ix) संयमात् *saṁyamāt* = from the meditation on

(x) योगी *yogi* = the yogī

(o) भूतजय: *bhūta-jayaḥ* =

(xi) भूतेषु *bhūteṣu* = on the pańca-mahā-bhūtas, on tha five basic-elements

(xii) विजय: *vijayaḥ* = वशीकरणम्, स्वायत्तीकरणम्, जय: control over

(xiii) प्राप्नोति *prāpnoti* = attains

From the meditation on the five states viz. (i) the five tangible orders namely hearing, touch, form, taste and smell of the beings, (ii) the five intangible orders namely solidity, fluidity, warmth, density and span (iii) the subtle elements i.e. the brain interpretive centers (iv) the three *sat, rajas* and *tamas guṇas* (v) and the motive, the *yogī* achieves control over the *pańca-mahā-bhūtas* (five basic-elements).

Comments : The knowledge of attaining success over the five basic elements comes from the meditation on above mentioned five states.

3.45 ततोऽणिमादिप्रादुर्भाव: कायसम्पत्तद्धर्मानभिघातश्च ।

tato'ṇimādiprādurbhāvaḥ kāyasampattaddharmānabhighātaśca

(tato-'ṇimādi-prādurbhāvaḥ kāya-sampat-tad-dharmānabhighātaḥ ća)

(i) तत: *tatḥ* = तस्मात् भूतजयात् = from that control over the mahā-bhūtas

(o) अणिमा–आदि–प्रादुर्भाव: *aṇimādi-prādurbhāvaḥ* =

(ii) अणिमा आदि *aṇimā-ādi* = capacity to miniaturize oneself, to make body very light, to make body very large, to make body very heavy, to obtai objects by thinking alone, to fulfill desires by imagination alone, to control five elements, to transform objects, etc.

(iii) अष्ट–सिद्धिनां प्रादुर्भाव: *aṣṭa siddhānām prādurbhāvaḥ* = उदय:, विकाश:, विकास:, उत्पत्ति: achieving of eight successes

(iv) भवति *bhavati* = becomes, occurs, happens, becomes possible

(v) एवं च *avam cha* = and

(o) कायसम्पत् *kāya-sampat* =

(vi) काय *kāya* = देहस्य. शरीरस्य of the body

(vii) सम्पत् *sampat* = सम्पदा, धनम्, संपत्तिः, वैभवः, ऐश्वर्यम्, समृद्धिः enrichment

(viii) भवति *bhavati* = becomes, occurs, happens, takes place

(ix) तथा च *tathā cha* = and

(o) तत्-धर्म-अनभिघातः *tad-dharmānabhighātaḥ* =

(x) ततः *tataḥ* = thereby

(xi) धर्मस्य *dharmasya* = सदाचारस्य, सच्चरित्र्यस्य, सौजन्यस्य, भद्रतायाः of righteousness

(xii) अभिघातः *abhighātaḥ* = घातः, हानिः, क्षयः, नाशः downfall

(xiii) अपि न भवति *api na bhavati* = also does not occur

📖 **From that control over the *mahā-bhūtas*, the *yogī* is able to achieve eight successes namely (i) capacity to miniaturize oneself, (ii) to make body very light, (iii) to make body very large, (iv) to make body very heavy, (v) to obtain objects by thinking alone, (vi) to fulfill desires by imagination alone, (vii) to control five elements, (viii) to transform objects, etc. and enrichment of the body occurs; and thereby downfall of one's righteousness does not occur.**

कायसम्पत् ।

kāyāsampat

77. Beauty and Strength

3.46 रूपलावण्यबलवज्रसंहननत्वानि कायसम्पत् ।

rūpalāvaṇyabalavajrasam̐hananatvāni kāyasampat

(rūpa-lāvaṇya-bala-vajra-sam̐hananatvāni kāya-sampat)

(o) रूप-लावण्य-बल-वज्र-संहननत्वानि *rūpa-lāvaṇya-bala-vajra-sam̐hananatvāni* =

(i) रूपस्य *rūpasya* = स्वरूपस्य, छवेः of form

(ii) लावण्यस्य *lāvaṇyasya* = सौन्दर्यस्य, कान्तेः, चारुतायाः beauty

(iii) बलस्य *balasya* = शक्तेः, प्रभावस्य, सामर्थ्यस्य strength

(iv) वज्रस्य *vajrasya* = काठिन्यस्य, दृढतायाः, धैर्यस्य of courage

(v) शरीरे संहननत्वानि *śarīre saṁhananatvāni* = देहे सम्बद्धत्वानि collection in the body

(vi) काय-सम्पत् *kāya-sampat* = देहस्य धनानि the wealth, treasures of the body

(vii) भवन्ति *bhavanti* = are, become

📖 **Collection of form, beauty, strength and courage, are the treasures of the body.**

इन्द्रियजयः ।

indriyavijayaḥ

78. Conquering Organs

3.47 ग्रहणस्वरूपास्मितान्वयार्थवत्त्वसंयमादिन्द्रियजयः ।

grahaṇasvarūpāsmitānvayārthavattvasaṁyamādindriyavijayaḥ

(grahaṇa-svarūpāsmitānvayārthavattva-saṁyamād-indriya-vijayaḥ)

(o) ग्रहण-स्वरूप-अस्मिता-अन्वय-अर्थवत्त्व-संयमात् *grahaṇa-svarūpa-asmitā-anvaya-arthavattva-saṁyamāt* =

(i) ग्रहणं *grahaṇam* = स्वीकरणम्, लभनम्, अधिगमनम्, प्रापणम् the state of mind while relishing senses

(ii) स्वरूपं *svarūpam* = स्वभावः, रूपम्, प्रकृतिः natural inborn state of mind

(iii) अस्मिता *asmitā* = अस्मि इति भावः, आत्मनः च बुद्धेः भेदः, आत्मानं च बुद्धिं च अभेदवत् मननम्, अहङ्कारः illusion of indifference

(iv) अन्वयः *anvayaḥ* = गुणत्रयस्य प्रभावः, सत्-रजस्-तमसादि गुणप्रभावः the influence of three guṇas

(v) अर्थवत्त्वं *arthavattvam* = गूढार्थः, तात्पर्यम्, निरूपणम् understanding the inner meaning

(vi) आदिनां वृत्तीनां *āfi vṛttinām* = the five states namely

(vii) संयमात् *saṁyamāt* = निग्रहात्, संयमनात् by meditating on

(viii) इन्द्रियविजय: *indriya-vijayaḥ* = इन्द्रियस्य जय:, इन्द्रियनिग्रह:, इन्द्रियवशीकरणम् control over his organs

(ix) लभते *labhate* = the yogī achieves

📖 **By meditating on the five states namely (i) the state of mind while relishing senses, (ii) natural inborn state of mind (iii) illusion of indifference (iv) the influence of three guṇas (v) understanding the inner meaning, the *yogī* achieves control over his organs.**

✍ Comments : The knowledge to control one's organs comes from the meditation on the above mentioned five states.

3.48 तत: मनोजवित्वं विकरणभाव: प्रधानजयश्च ।

tataḥ manojavitvam vikaraṇabhāvaḥ pradhāna-jayaśca

(tataḥ mano-javitvam vikaraṇa-bhāvaḥ pradhāna-jayaḥ ća)

(i) तत: *tataḥ* = इन्द्रियेषु विजयं प्राप्त्वा = after, by achieving control over organs

(o) मनोजवित्वम् *mano-javitvam* =

(ii) मनस: सदृशं *manasaḥ sadṛśam* = like the mind

(iii) जवित्वं *javitvam* = गति:, चालना, वेग:, जव: motion, speed

(iv) च *cha* = and

(v) विकरण-भाव: *vikaraṇa-bhāvah* = विदेह-वृत्ति-लाभ: capacity to experience senses

(vi) शरीरातीत-विषय-प्राप्ति: *śarīrātīta-viṣaya-prāptiḥ* without the use of organs

(vii) प्रधान-जय: *pradhāna-jayaḥ* = प्रकृते: विकारेषु विजय:, गुणेषु तटस्थता and control over nature

(viii) प्राप्यते *prapyate* = also comes, he attains

📖 **By achieving control over organs, comes speed like the mind, and capacity to** experience senses without the use of organs and comes control over nature.

3.49 सत्त्वपुरुषान्यताख्यातिमात्रस्य सर्वभावाधिष्ठातृत्वं सर्वज्ञातृत्वमं च ।

sattvapuruṣānyatākhyātimātrasya sarvabhāvādhiṣṭhātṛtvam sarvajñātṛtvam ća

(sattva-puruṣānyatākhyāti-mātrasya sarva-bhāvādhiṣṭhātṛtvam sarva-jñātṛtvam ća)

(o) सत्त्व-पुरुष-अन्यता-ख्याति-मात्रस्य *sattva-puruṣānyatākhyāti-mātrasya* =

(i) प्रकृति-पुरुषयो *pṛkriti-puruṣahyoḥ* = of pṛkriti and puruṣa

(ii) भिन्नतायाः ज्ञानम् *bhinnatāyāḥ jñānam* = the understanding of the difference between

(o) सर्व-भाव-अधिष्ठातृत्वम् *sarva-bhāvādhiṣṭhātṛtvam* =

(iii) सर्वेषु *sarveṣu* = in all

(iv) भावेषु *bhāveṣu* = सत्तासु, वृत्तिषु sentiments (see 2.34)

(v) अध्यक्षतायाः *adhyakṣatāyāḥ* = अनुशास्तृत्वस्य of control over

(vi) ज्ञानं *jñānam* = understanding

(vii) च *cha* = and

(viii) सर्व-ज्ञातृत्वम् *sarva-jñātṛtvam* = सर्वज्ञत्वं, अपरज्ञानम् omniscience

(ix) लभते *labhate* = such yogī achieves

📖 **Such *yogī* achieves (i) the understanding of the difference between *pṛkritiḥ* and *puruṣaḥ* and (ii) of the control over all sentiments and he attains omniscience.**

कैवल्यम् ।

kaivalyam

79. Liberation

3.50 तद्वैराग्यादपि दोषबीजक्षये कैवल्यम् ।

tadvairāgyādapi doṣabījakṣaye kaivalyam

(tat-vairāgyād-api doṣa-bīja-kṣaye kaivalyam)

(i) तत् *tat* = तेभ्य:, ज्ञानत्रयेभ्य:, तटस्थताया:, वैराग्यात् from the non-attachment of these three faculties

(ii) दोष-बीज-क्षये *doṣa-bīja-kṣaye* = दोषस्य बीजस्य नाशात् as a result of the removal of the source of obstacle (see 2.33, 34 above).

(iii) कैवल्यम् *kaivalyam* = असंसृष्टता, मुक्ति:, मोक्ष:, निर्वाणम् everlasting escape

(iv) प्राप्यते *prāpyate* = (the yogī) attains

📖 **From the non-attachment of the three faculties of (i) indifference, (ii) non-attachment, and (iii) asceticism, as a result of the removal of the source of obstacle, the *yogī* attains everlasting escape.**

✍ Comments : Everlasting escape from the cycle of the birth, death and re-birth is *kaivalyam.*

3.51 स्थान्युपनिमन्त्रेण सङ्गस्मयाकरणं पुनरनिष्टप्रसङ्गात् ।

sthānyupanimantreṇa saṅgasmayākaraṇam punaraniṣṭaprasaṅgāt

(sthāny-upanimantreṇa saṅga-smayākaraṇam punar-aniṣṭa-prasaṅgāt)

(o) स्थानि-उपनिमन्त्रेण *sthāni-upanimantreṇa* =

(i) तत: *tataḥ* = thereafter

(ii) ऊर्ध्व-लोकस्य निमन्त्रणेन *ūrdhva-lokasya nimantreṇa* = with the invitation from the liberation

(iii) स: योगी *saḥ yogi* = that yogī

(iv) सङ्ग-स्मय-अकरणम् *saṅga-smaya-akaraṇam* = न सङ्गं न अहङ्कारं कुर्यात् should not possess ego

(v) पुनर्-अनिष्ट-प्रसङ्गात् *punar-aaniṣṭa-prasaṅgāt* = नो चेत् पुन: otherwise again

(vi) अनिष्ट: *punar-aniṣṭa* = अनपेक्षित:, अवाञ्छित:, अनभिलषित: undesired

(vii) प्रसङ्ग: *prasaṅga* = संभव:, अवसर:, घटना thing

(viii) संभवेत् *sambhavet* = may occur

📖 **Thereafter, with the invitation from the liberation, that *yogī* should not possess ego, otherwise, again undesired thing may occur.**

✍ Comments : After attaining *kaivalya*, one should not possess ego. It will bring you back in the birth-cycle.

3.52 क्षणतत्क्रमयोः संयमाद्विविवेकजं ज्ञानम् ।

kṣaṇatatkramayoḥ saṁyamādvivekajam jñānam

(kṣaṇa-tat-kramayoḥ saṁyamād-vivekajam jñānam)

(o) क्षण–तत्–क्रमयोः *kṣaṇa-tat-kramayoḥ* =

(i) *kṣaṇa tasya* क्षणस्य, मुहूर्तस्य, निमेषस्य, अवसरस्य तस्य on that time, on time

(ii) क्रमस्य *kramasy* = अनुक्रमस्य, विन्यासस्य, विरचनस्य of sequence

(iii) संयमात् *saṁyamāt* = निग्रहात् by meditating on

(iv) विवेकजम् *vivekajam* = बुद्धिजातम् borne out of thinking

(v) ज्ञानं *jñānam* = understanding

(vi) लभते *labhate* = comes, the yogī earns.

📖 **By meditating on the time sequence, the *yogī* earns understanding borne out of thinking.**

✍ Comments : The knowledge of universal understanding comes from the meditation on the time sequence.

3.53 जातिलक्षणदेशैरन्यतानवच्छेदात्तुल्ययोस्ततः प्रतिपत्तिः ।

jātilakṣaṇadeśairanyānavacchedāttulyayohstataḥ pratipattiḥ

(jāti-lakṣaṇa-deśair-anyānavacchedāt-tulyayohs-tataḥ pratipattiḥ)

(i) ततः *tataḥ* = तस्मात् विवेकज्ञानात् with such understanding

(o) जाति-लक्षण-देशैः *jāti-lakṣaṇa-deśaiḥ* =

(ii) जातिः *jātiḥ* = जन्म birth

(iii) लक्षणं *lakṣaṇam* = चारित्र्य, अभिज्ञानम् signs, appearance

(iv) देशैः *deśaiḥ* = स्थानैः = and place

(v) अन्यता-अनवच्छेदात् *anyatā-anavaććhedāt* = अभेदवत् स्थितेः कारणात्, तटस्थतायाः as a result of indifference to

(vi) तुल्ययोः *tulyayoḥ* = द्वन्द्व-भावे समानता of equanimity in the pairs opposite sentiments

(vii) प्रतिपत्तिः *pratipattiḥ* = उपलब्धिः, प्राप्तिः attainment

(viii) भवति *bhavati* = becomes, occurs, happens, takes place

📖 **With such understanding, as a result of indifference to birth, appearance, and place, occurs attainment of equanimity in the pairs of opposite sentiments.**

✍ Comments : The universal understanding gives indifference to the pairs of the opposites.

3.54 तारकं सर्वविषयं सर्वथाविषयमक्रममं चेति विवेकजं ज्ञानम् ।

tārakam sarvaviśayam sarvathāviṣayamakramam ćeti vivekajam jñānam

(tārakam sarva-viśayam sarvathā-viṣayam-akramam ćeti vivekajam jñānam)

(i) तारकं *tārakam* = त्रातरं, उद्धर्तारम्, तारणकर्तारम्, परित्रातरम् the savior

(ii) सर्व-विषयम् *sarva-viśayam* = सर्वज्ञं, सर्वविदम्, कृत्स्नज्ञम् the all-knower

(iii) सर्वथा-विषयम् = सर्व-प्रकारेण च and in all way

(iv) अक्रमम् *akramam* = इति विवेकात् जनितं ज्ञानं, सदसज्ज्ञानम् understanding of borne out of thinking

(v) च इति *cha iti* = thus

(vi) वर्तते *vatrate* = is

📖 **The savior and the all-knower in all way is the understanding of borne out of thinking.**

✍ Comments : The universal understanding is the savior.

3.55 सत्त्वपुरुषयोः शुद्धिसाम्ये कैवल्यम् ।

sattvapuruṣayoḥ śuddhisāmye kaivalyam

(sattva-puruṣayoḥ śuddhi-sāmye kaivalyam)

(i) सत्त्व-पुरुषयोः *sattva-puruṣayoḥ* = प्रकृति-पुरुषयोः, गुण-आत्मनोः of prakṛtiḥ and puruṣaḥ and the guṇas and ātmā

(ii) शुद्धि-साम्ये *śuddhi-sāmye* = साम्य-भावेन with equanimity

(iii) यदा *yadā* = when

(iv) मात्र शुद्धिः *mātra shuddhiḥ* = यथार्थता clarity of understanding

(v) भवति *bhavati* = becomes, occurs, happens

(vi) तदा *tadā* = then

(vii) 'कैवल्यम्' *kaivalyam* = असंसृष्टता, मुक्तिः, मोक्षः liberation, emancipation

(viii) आयाति *āyāti* = comes

📖 **When clarity of understanding of *prakṛtiḥ* and *puruṣaḥ* and the *guṇas* and the *ātmā* occurs with equanimity, then comes liberation.**

✍ Comments : Liberation comes fro the understanding of the *purusha, prikriti, gunas* and the *atma.* (Gita 4:9)

4. कैवल्यपादः ।

kaivalyapādaḥ

सिद्धिः ।

siddhiḥ

80. Success

4.1 जन्मौषधिमन्त्रतपःसमाधिजाः सिद्धयः ।

janmauṣadhimantratapaḥsamādhijāḥ siddhayaḥ

(janm-auṣadhi-mantra-tapaḥ-samādhijāḥ siddhayaḥ)

(o) जन्म–औषधि–मन्त्र–तपः–समाधिजाः *janm-auṣadhi-mantra-tapaḥ-samādhihāḥ* =

(i) जन्मजा *janmajā* = जन्मात् जायते या borne out of birth

(ii) औषधिजा *auṣadhijā* = औषधात् जायते या borne out of a remedy

(iii) मन्त्रजा *mantrajā* = मन्त्रात् जायते या borne out incantation

(iv) तपःजा *tapaḥjā* = तपसः जायते या borne out of austerity

(v) समाधिजा च *samādhijā cha* = समाधेः जायते या and borne out of meditation

(vi) इति पञ्च *iti pañcha* = these five

(vii) 'सिद्धयः' *siddhayaḥ* = 'siddhis,' successes, achievements

(viii) सन्ति *santi* = are

📖 **(i) Borne out of birth, (ii) borne out of a remedy, (iii) borne out incantation, (iv) borne out of austerity and (v) borne out of meditation, are five *siddhis* (successes).**

✍ Comments : Successes are of five types shown above.

जात्यन्तरम् ।

jātyantaram

81. Change of Genera

4.2 जात्यन्तरपरिणामः प्रकृत्यापूरात् ।

jātyantarapariṇāmaḥ prakṛtyāpurāt

(jātyantara-pariṇāmaḥ prakṛtyā-purāt)

(i) जाति-अन्तर-परिणामः *jāti-antara-pariṇāmaḥ* = जन्मनां अन्तरस्य परिणामः, जन्मनां अन्तरस्य फलम्, जन्मनां अन्तरेषु परिवर्तनम्, जन्मजन्मनि रूपान्तरम् transmigration

(o) प्रकृति-आपूरात् *prakṛtyā-purāt* =

(ii) प्रकृतेः *prakṛteḥ* = of prakṛti

(iii) आपूरात् *āpurāt* = पूर्णत्वात्, साकल्यात् from the imbalance to balance

(iv) भवति *bhavati* = becomes, occurs, happens, takes place

🕮 **Transmigration occurs as a result of the imbalance of the *prakṛti.***

✍ Comments : Balance state of the elements is *prakriti*. From an imbalance in the *prakriti* occurs transmigration to bring back the balance.

4.3 निमित्तमप्रयोजकं प्रकृतीनां वरणभेदस्तु ततः क्षेत्रिकवत् ।

nimittamaprayojakam prakṛtinān varaṇabhedastu tataḥ kṣetrikavat

(nimittam-aprayojakam prakṛtinām varaṇa-bhedastu tataḥ kṣetrika-vat)

(i) निमित्तम् *nimittam* = जन्म-औषधि-मन्त्र-तपः-समाधि-आदीनि निमित्तानि, कारणानि the causes such as birth, remedy, incantations, austerity, meditation etc.

(ii) प्रकृतीनाम् *prakṛtinām* = प्रकृतेः तत्त्वानाम् for the functioning of prakṛtiḥ

(iii) अप्रयोजकम् *aprayojakam* = प्रयोजनानि न सन्ति are not the reasons

(iv) तु *tu* = परन्तु but

(v) ते ततः *te tataḥ* = they thereby

(o) वरण-भेदः *varaṇa-bhedaḥ* =

(vi) वरणस्य *varaṇasya* = आवरणस्य the hurdle

(vii) भेदः *bhedaḥ* = अपसारणम्, निःसारणम्, स्थानभेदः removal of

(viii) क्षेत्रिकवत् *kṣetrika-vat* = कृषकवत् like a farmer

(viii) कुर्वन्ति *kurvanti* = do the function of

📖 **The causes such as birth, remedy, incantations, austerity, meditation etc. are not the reasons <u>for the functioning</u> of *prakṛtiḥ*, but they thereby do the function of removal of the hurdle, like a farmer does in the field.**

✍ Comments : The birth, austerity, meditation, etc. are not the reasons for the *prikriti*.

अस्मिता ।

asmitā

82. Unification of Vision and Visibility

4.4 निर्माणचित्ताण्यस्मितामात्रात् ।

nirmāṇachittānyasmitāmātrāt *(nirmāṇa-chittānya-smitā-mātrāt)*

(o) निर्माण-चित्तानि *nirmāṇa-chittā* =

(i) निर्माणानि *nirmāṇānī* = निर्माणानि, निर्मितानि, आधितानि, संपादितानि, रचितानि the fabricated

(ii) चित्तानि *chittāni* = वृत्तयः, मतयः, अवधानानि, मनोयोगाः, धारणाः, अवेक्षाः thoughts, minds

(iii) अस्मिता-मात्रात् *a-smitā-mātrāt* = केवलम् अस्मितायाः क्लेशभेदात् only due to the illusion of difference (see 2.3 above)

(iv) भवन्ति *bhavanti* = are

📖 **The <u>fabricated thoughts</u> are only due to the illusion of difference.**

✍ Comments : The illusion of indifference is *asmita.*

4.5 प्रवृत्तिभेदे प्रयोजकं चित्तमेकमनेकेषाम् ।

pravṛttibhede prayojakam chittamekamanekeṣām

(pravṛtti-bhede prayojakam chittam-ekam-anekeṣām)

(i) अनेकेषाम् *anekeṣām* = बहुनां of many

(ii) चित्तानां *chittānām* = वृत्तीनाम्, मतीनाम्, अवधानानाम्, मनोयोगानाम्, धारणानाम्, अवेक्षाणाम् of thoughts

(iii) प्रवृत्तिभेदे *pravṛtti-bhede* = नाना प्रवृत्तिषु in various ways

(iv) प्रयोजकं *prayojakam* = नियोजकं, उपयोक्ता प्रेरकः, व्यवस्थापकः, अनुष्ठाता the assigner

(v) चित्तम् *chittam* = अन्तःकरणं, हृदयं, मनः, चेतः the mind

(vi) एकम् *ekam* = एकमात्रम् एव only

(vii) भवति *bhavati* = is, becomes, occurs, happens

📖 **The <u>assigner</u> of many thoughts in various ways is the mind only.**

✍ Comments : The mind is the assigner of thoughts.

4.6 तत्र ध्यानजमनाशयम् ।

tatra dhyānajamanāśayam *(tatra dhyānajam-anāśayam)*

(i) तत्र *tatra* = तस्मिन् चित्तेषु = among those thoughts

(ii) ध्यानजम् *dhyānajam* = ध्यान-जनितं, अवधानजन्यम्, मनोयोगजम्, समाधिजनितम् the one borne out of meditation

(iii) अन्-आशयम् *an-āśayam* = कर्म-संस्कार-रहितं without impression of karma

(iv) भवति *bhavati* = is, becomes, occurs, happens

Among those thoughts, the one borne out of meditation is without impression of *karma*.

Comments : The thought borne out of meditation is without impression of *karma*.

कर्म ।

karma

83. Deed

4.7 कर्माशुक्लाकृष्णं योगिनस्त्रिविधमितरेषाम् ।

karmāśuklākṛṣṇam yoginastrividhamitareṣām

(karmā-śuklā-kṛṣṇam yoginaḥ-tri-vidham-itareṣām)

(i) योगिन: कर्म *yoginaḥ karma* = the karmas of a yogī are

(o) अशुक्ल-अकृष्णम् *aśuklā-akṛṣṇam* =

(ii) अशुक्लम् *aśuklam* = अ-पाप-कारकं without the impression of righteous impression

(iii) अकृष्णं च *akṛṣṇam cha* = अ-पुण्य-कारकं and without the impression of sin (see 1.24↑)

(iv) इति कर्म-संस्कार-शून्यौ *iti karma-saṁskāra-shūnyau* = in this way without either of the two impression

(v) भवत: *bhavataḥ* = are

(vi) इतरेषाम् *itareṣām* = अयोगिनां कर्म work of other people

(vii) शुक्लं *śuklam* = पाप-कारकं without sin causing

(viii) कृष्णं *kṛṣṇam* = पुण्य-कारकं without merit causing

(ix) मिश्रं *miśram* = पुण्यं च पापं च कारकं sin causing or merit causing

(x) इति त्रिविधानि *iti tri-vidhāni* = in these three ways

(xi) भवन्ति *bhavanti* = they are

📖 **The *karmas* of the *yogī* are (i) without the impression of sin and (ii) without the impression of righteousness. In this way, they are, without either impression. Of other people, they are of three ways, (i) without sin causing, (ii) without merit causing and (iii) sin causing or merit causing.**

✍ Comments : See Gītā 18:12

फलम् ।

phalam

84. Fruit, Result

4.8 ततस्तद्विपाकानुगुणानामेवाभिव्यक्तिर्वासनानाम् ।

tatastadvipākānuguṇānāmevābhivyaktirvāsanāmām

(tataḥ-tad-vipākānuguṇānām-evābhivyaktir-vāsanāmām)

(i) ततः *tataḥ* = तस्मात् त्रिविध-कर्मात् from those three types of karmas of the non-yogīs

(ii) तत्-विपाक-अनुगुणानाम् *tat-vipākānuguṇānām* = तेषां फल-भोगानुकुलम् according to the distined fruits of those karmas

(iii) एव *eva* = केवलं, मात्र only

(iv) वासनानाम् *vāsanāmām* = कामनानां, प्रत्याशानाम्, वाञ्छानाम् of desires

(v) अभिव्यक्तिः *abhivyaktiḥ* = स्वरूपं, प्रकटनम् expression

(vi) भवति *bhavati* = is, becomes, occurs, happens

📖 **From those three types of *karmas* of the non-*yogīs*, occurs expression of desires, according to the destined fruits of those *karmas*.**

✍ Comments : For the non-yogis, the *karmas* yield three types of destined fruits.

4.9 जातिदेशकालव्यवहितानामप्यानन्तर्यं स्मृतिसंस्कारयोरेकरूपत्वात् ।

jātideśakālavyavahitāmāmapyānantaryam smṛtisaṁskārayorekarūpatvāt

(jāti-deśa-kāla-vyavahitāmām-apyānantaryam smṛti-saṁskārayor-eka-rūpatvāt)

(o) जाति-देश-काल-व्यवहितानाम् *jāti-deśa-kāla-vyavahitāmām* =

(i) जाति *jāti* = जन्म birth

(ii) देश *deśa* = स्थान place

(iii) काल *kāla* = समय time

(iv) आदिनां *ādinām* = etc.

(v) व्यवहितानां *vyavahitāmām* = व्यवधानानाम्, असन्निहितानाम्, अन्तराणाम् of such an interposition as

(o) स्मृति-संस्कारयो: *smṛti-saṁskārayoḥ* =

(vi) स्मृते: च *smṛteḥ cha* = remembrance and

(vii) संस्कारस्य *saṁskārasya* = of previous impression

(viii) एक-रूपत्वात् *eka-rūpatvāt* = साम्यात्, अभिन्नत्वात् oneness

(ix) आनन्तर्यम् *ānantaryam* = अन्तरं, कर्म-संस्कारेषु चित्तावक्षेप:, व्यवधानम् difference

(x) न विद्यते *na vidyate* = does not exist

📖 **Of such an interposition as birth, place or time etc. there is no difference in impact on *karma*, because of the oneness of remembrance and impact of previous impressions.**

✍ Comments : The impressions of *Karma* are not affected by birth, place or time.

4.10 तासामनादित्वं चाशिषो नित्यत्वात् ।

tāsāmanāditvam cāśiṣo nityatvāt *(tāsām-anāditvam cāśiṣo nityatvāt)*

(i) तासाम् *tāsām* = तासां वासनानां, कामनानाम् of those desires

(ii) अनादित्वम् *anāditvam* = आरम्भ-शून्यता, नित्यत्वम् the perpetuity

(iii) यत: *yataḥ* = because, due to

(iv) भूतानां आशिष: *bhutānām āśiṣaḥ* = आशास्यम्, हितोद्देश: interest in self preservation of the beings

(v) नित्यत्वात् *nityatvāt* = अनादि-कालत: from perpetuity

(vi) एव वर्तते *eva vartate* = exists

📖 **The perpetuity of those desires is due to interest of the beings in self preservation exists from perpetuity.**

✍ Comments : Perpetuity of desires in the beings comes from their interest of self preservation.

4.11 हेतुफलाश्रयालन्बनै: संगृहीतत्वादेषामभावे तदभाव: ।

hetuphalāśrayālambanaiḥ sanhṛhitatvādeṣāmabhāve tadabhāvaḥ

(hetu-phal-āśray-ālambanaiḥ sanhṛhitatvād-eṣām-abhāve tad-abhāvaḥ)

(o) हेतु-फल-आश्रय-आलन्बनै: *hetu-phal-āśray-ālambanaiḥ* =

(i) वासनानां हेतुना *vāsanānām hetunā* = अविद्यादि-क्लेशै: with the aim of fulfilling desires

(ii) वासनानां फलेन *vāsanānām phalena* = पुनर्जन्मादि-भोगै: with the experience of desires in the previous births

(iii) वासनानां आश्रयेण *vāsanānām āśrayeṇa* with the attachment of desires

(iv) वासनानां आलम्बेन *vāsanānām ālambena* = शब्दादि-विषयै: with the senses of the desires

(v) संगृहीतत्वात् *sanhṛhitatvāt* = वासनानं संग्रहं भवति occurs accumulation os desires

(vi) परन्तु एषाम् *parantu eṣām* = उपरोक्तानां चतुर्णाम् अभावे, अभावात्, अविद्यमानताया: but without the presence of these four precursors of desires

(vii) तद्-अभाव: *tad-abhāvaḥ* = तासाम् वासनानाम् अभाव: अविद्यमानता absence of those desires also

(viii) विद्यते *vidyate* = occurs

📖 **With the (i) aim of fulfilling desires, (ii) with the experience of desires in the previous births, (iii) with the attachment of desires, and (iv) with the senses of the desires, occurs accumulation of desires. But without the presence of these four precursors of desires, absence of those desires also occurs.**

✍ Comments : The accumulation of desires through lives occurs as a result of the above given four precursors.

गुणधर्माः ।

guṇadharmāḥ

85. Nature and Properties

4.12 अतीतानागतं स्वरूपतोऽस्त्यध्वभेदाद्धर्माणाम् ।

atītānāgatam svarūpato'styadhvabhedāddharmāṇām

(atītān-āgatam svarūpato-'styadhva-bhedad-dharmāṇām)

(i) धर्माणाम् *dharmāṇām* = गुणानाम्, नित्यगुणानाम्, स्वभावानाम्, वस्तूनां of the things

(ii) अध्वभेदात् *adhva-bhedat* = as a result of the nature

(iii) अध्वनः *adhvanaḥ* मार्गस्य, नियमस्य, अन्तरस्य, वृत्तेः, समयस्य, वातावरणस्य, प्रक्रियायाः of time

(iv) भेदात् *bhedat* = अन्तरात्, भिन्नतायाः, पृथक्त्वात्, परत्वात् difference in

(o) अतीत-अनागतम् *atītān-āgatam* =

(v) अतीतः *atītaḥ* = भूतः, भूतकालः the past

(vi) अनागतः च *ān-āgataḥ cha* = भविष्यः च and the future

(vii) धर्मः *dharmaḥ* = स्वरूपम् = nature

(viii) स्वरूपतः *svarūpataḥ* = स्वस्य बीज-रूपेण, स्वभावानुसारेण according to its own make up

(ix) सर्वेऽपि वस्तु-गुणधर्माः *sarve-api vastu-guṇa-dharmāḥ* = the nature of every thing

(x) सन्ति *santi* = are, is

📖 **As a result of time there is difference in the nature of the things. The past and the future nature of every thing is according to its own make up.**

✍ Comments : The difference in the nature of beings is due to the difference in the three times.

4.13 ते व्यक्तसूक्ष्मा गुणात्मनः ।

te vyaktasūkṣmā guṇātmanaḥ *(te vyakta-sūkṣmā guṇātmanaḥ)*

(i) ते *te* = ते सर्वे धर्माः, गुणाः, स्वभावाः All those natures of things

(o) व्यक्त–सूक्ष्माः *vyakta-sūkṣmā* =

(ii) व्यक्त–रूपेण *vyakta-rūpeṇa* = गोचर, प्रकट, विद्यमान, स्फुट, विशद, प्रत्यक्ष, प्रकाशित apparent

(iii) वा सूक्ष्म *va sūkṣmarūprṇa* = बीज, अगोचर, अप्रकट, अविद्यमान, अप्रत्यक्ष, अप्रकाशित or non-apparent

(o) गुण–आत्मनः *guṇātmanaḥ* =

(iv) आत्मनः *ātmanaḥ* = स्वीय, स्वकीय, आत्मीय their own

(v) गुण–रूपेण *guṇarūprṇa* = in the form of three guṇas

(vi) सन्ति *santi* = are

📖 **All those natures of things, either apparent or non-apparent, are in the form of their own three *guṇas*.**

✍ Comments : The nature of things id due to their *gunas*.

4.14 परिणामैकत्वाद्वस्तुतत्त्वम् ।

pariṇāmaiktvādvastutattvam *(pariṇām-aiktvād-vastu-tattvam)*

(o) परिणाम–एकत्वात् *pariṇāma-ektvād* =

(i) परिणामस्य *pariṇamasya* = फलस्य, सिद्धेः, निष्पत्तेः in the effect of the guṇas

(ii) एकत्वात् *ektvāt* = एकतायाः, साम्यात् from the uniformity

(o) वस्तु-तत्त्वम् *vastu-tattvam* =

(iii) वस्तुनः *vastunaḥ* = द्रव्यस्य, भूतस्य of things

(iv) तत्त्वं *tattvam* = तथ्यम्, यथार्थः, सत्यता, सत्ता, सारः existance

(v) विद्यते *vidyate* = there is

📖 **There is uniformity in the effect of the *guṇas*, and thus there is such uniform existence of things.**

✍ Comments : The uniformity of the effects of the *gunas* is the reason for the uniformity in the nature of the beings.

पन्थाः ।

panthāḥ

86. Mode, way

4.15 वस्तुसाम्ये चित्तभेदात्तयोर्विभक्तः पन्थाः ।

vastusāmye chittabhedāttayorvibhaktaḥ panthāḥ

(vastu-sāmye chitta-bhedāt-tayor-vibhaktaḥ panthāḥ)

(i) वस्तु-साम्ये *vastu-sāmye* = वस्तुनः एकत्वे अपि even in the apparent uniformity of things

(ii) चित्त-भेदात् *chitta-bhedāt* = चित्तस्य, मनसः, चेतसः due to their distinctness from mind

(iii) तयोः *tayoḥ* = वृत्तीनां, अवस्थानाम्, स्वभावानाम्चित्त-वस्तुनोः of their nature, of the thing and mind

(iv) भेदात् *bhedāt* = भिन्नतायाः, पृथक्त्वात् difference

(v) पन्थाः *panthāḥ* = मार्गः, वर्त्म, चयनम्, नियमः, विधः the mode of behavior

(vi) विभक्तः *vibhaktaḥ* = भिन्नः, विभिन्नः, पृथक् different

(vii) अस्ति *asti* = is

📖 **Even in the apparent uniformity of things, there is difference in their nature** due to their distinctness from mind. The way of behavior of the things and the mind is different.**

✍ Comments : However, the difference in their minds, causes the distinctness among the apparently uniform beings.

4.16 न चैकचित्ततन्त्रं वस्तु तदप्रमाणकं तदा किं स्यात् ।

na ćaikaćittatantram vastu tadpramāṇakam tadā kim syāt

(na ćaika-ćitta-tantram vastu tad-apramāṇakam tadā kim syāt)

(i) च *cha* = अपि च, अपरं च, अधिकः, भूयः again

(ii) वस्तु *vastu* = दृश्य-पदार्थः any apparent thing

(o) एक-चित्त-तन्त्रम् *ek-ćitta-tantram* =

(iii) किमपि एकेन *kimapi ekena* = with any one

(iv) वस्तुनः तन्त्रेण *vastunaḥ tantreṇa* = अधीनम्, आधारेण, सूत्रेण, शासनेन, मन्त्रेण physical principle

(v) न *na* = न विद्यते = does not exist or behave

(vi) यतः *yataḥ* = because

(o) तत् अ-प्रमाणकं *tat apramāṇakam* =

(vii) यदा तत् वस्तु *yadā tat vastu* = when a thing

(viii) चित्तस्य *chittasya* = मनसः, विचारस्य, दृष्टेः, चेतसः of mind

(ix) प्रमाणकं *pramāṇakam* = विषयः, हेतुः, साक्ष्यम्, इयत्ता the object

(x) न स्यात् *na syāt* = shall not be

(xi) किं स्यात् *kim syāt* = तदा किं भविष्यति? किं भवितुं शक्यते? then what will happen of the thing?

📖 **Again, any apparent thing does not exist or behave with any one physical principle. Because, when a thing shall not be the object of mind, then what will happen of the thing? (how will the thing be perceived)**

✍ Comments : The things do not exist with only one physical principle.

4.17 तदपरागापेक्षित्वाच्चित्तस्य वस्तु ज्ञाताज्ञातम् ।

tadaprāgāpekṣitvāććittasya vastu Jnãtājñātam

(tat-aprāgā-pekṣitvāć-ćittasya vastu Jnãtā-jñātam)

(i) चित्तस्य *ćittasya* = चेतसः, मनसः, दृष्टेः of the mind or vision

(o) तत्-उपराग-अपेक्षित्वात् *tat-aprāga-apekṣitvāt* =

(ii) तस्य *tat* = तस्य वस्तुनः = of a thing

(iii) अपरागस्य *aprāgasya* = विषयानुरागस्य contact of its sense

(iv) अपेक्षित्वात् *apekṣitvāt* = अनावश्यकत्वात्, अनभिष्टत्वात्, असम्बन्धात् without coming in contact

(v) वस्तु *vastu* = द्रव्यम्, दृश्य पदार्थः the thing

(o) ज्ञात-अज्ञातम् *jnãta-ajñātam* =

(vi) कदाचित् *kadāchit* = may be

(vii) ज्ञातं *Jnãtam* = परिचितम्, विदितम्, बुधितम् become known

(viii) वा कदाचित् *vā kadāchit* = or else

(ix) अज्ञातं *ajñānam* = अपरिचितम्, अविदितम्, अननुभूतम्, अगोचरम् not known

(x) वा वर्तते *vā vartate* = or becomes

📖 **When the sense of a thing comes in contact with the mind (or vision), the thing may become known; or else, without the contact, it does not become known.**

✍ Comments : A thing becomes known as a result of its contact with the mind.

4.18 सदा ज्ञाताश्चित्तवृत्तयस्तत्प्रभोः पुरुषस्यापरिणामित्वात् ।

sadā jñātāsćittavṛttayastatprabhoḥ puruṣasyāpariṇāmitvāt

(sadā jñātās-ćitta-vṛttayas-tat-prabhoḥ puruṣasyā-pariṇāmitvāt)

(o) तत्-प्रभोः *tat-prabhoḥ* =

(i) तत् वस्तु *tat vastu* = that thing itself

(ii) प्रभोः *prabhoḥ* = स्वामिनः, भगवतः of god

(iii) पुरुषस्य *puruṣasya* = ईशस्य, ईश्वरस्य of puruśa, of ātmā

(iv) परिणामित्वात् *pariṇāmitvāt* = परिणाम-तत्त्वं able to affect

(v) नास्ति *nāsti* = is not

(vi) ततः *tataḥ* = therefore

(vii) चित्त-वृत्तयः *ćitta-vṛttayaḥ* = the internal fluctuations of mind

(viii) सदा *sadā* = all time

(ix) ज्ञाताः *jñātāḥ* = the observers of

(x) सः *saḥ* = सः प्रभुः = that lord, that ātmā

(xi) प्राणिनां *prāṇinām* = of beings

(xii) चित्त-वृत्तीः *ćitta-vṛttīḥ* = अवस्थाः the states of mind

(xiii) पश्यन् अस्ति *paśyan asti* = is always observing

📖 **That external thing itself is not able to affect *ātmā*. Therefore, at all times *ātmā*, the observer of the internal fluctuations of mind, is always observing only the internal states of mind.**

✍ Comments : The things do not affect *atma*. The *atma* is an independent observer (Gita 6:31, 9:18).

4.19 न तत्स्वाभासं दृश्यत्वात् ।

na tatsvābhāsam dṛśyatvāt *(na tat-svābhāsam dṛśyatvāt)*

(i) तत् *tat* = तत् चित्तम् = that mind

(ii) स्व-आभासम् *svābhāsam* = स्वकाशं, आत्मज्ञम् self perceiver, able to perceive without contact

(iii) न *na* = नास्ति = not

(iv) यतः *yataḥ* = because

(v) दृश्यत्वात् *dṛśyatvāt* = तत् mind

(vi) दृश्यं *dṛśyam* = गोचरम् perceivable

(vii) अस्ति *asti* = is

📖 **That mind, is not able to perceive without contact, because the mind itself is perceivable.**

✍ Comments : Mind is not able to perceive without a contact.

4.20 एकसमये चोभयानवधारणम् ।

ekasamaye ćobhayānavadhāraṇam *(eka-samaye ćobhayān-avadhāraṇam)*

(i) च *cha* = तथा च and

(ii) एक-समये *eka-samaye* = युगपत्, एकपदे, एकत्र at one instant together

(o) उभय-अनवधारणम् *ubhaya-anvadhāraṇam* =

(iv) उभय *ubhaya* = चित्त-वस्तुनोः of both the ātmā and its object

(v) अवधारणं *avadhāraṇam* = बोधः, कल्पना, उपलब्धिः discernment

(vi) न भवति *na bhavati* = can not occur

📖 **And, discernment of both the *ātmā* and its object can not occur at one instant together.**

✍ Comments : The discernment of the *atma* and its object can not occur together.

4.21 चित्तान्तरदृश्ये बुद्धिबुद्धेरतिप्रसङ्गः स्मृतिसङ्करश्च ।

ćittāntaradṛśye buddhibuddheratiprasaṅgaḥ smṛtisaṅkarasća

(ćittāntara-dṛśye buddhi-buddher-atiprasaṅgaḥ smṛti-saṅkaraḥ ća)

(o) चित्त–अन्तर–दृश्ये *ćitta-antara-dṛśye* =

(ii) चित्तं *ćitta* = एकं चित्तम् one mind

(iii) अन्तरस्य *antarasya* = अन्यस्य चितस्य of another mind

(iv) दृश्ये *dṛśye* = लक्ष्ये, केन्द्रे, बिन्दौ focus of vision

(v) मत्वा *matvā* = having made, having considered

(vi) बुद्धि–बुद्धेः *buddhi-buddheḥ* = एकस्य चित्तस्य of one mind

(vii) अन्यं चित्तम् *anyam chittam* = other mind

(viii) अतिप्रसङ्गः *atiprasaṅgaḥ* = दृश्यं, लक्ष्यम्, केन्द्रबिन्दुः aim

(ix) भवति *bhavati* = becomes, occurs, happens

(x) च *cha* = and

(o) स्मृति–सङ्करः *smṛti-saṅkaraḥ* =

(xi) स्मृतयोः *smṛtayoḥ* = बुद्ध्योः of minds

(xii) सङ्करः *saṅkaraḥ* = मिलापः, मेलनम् mix up

(xiii) वर्तिष्यते *vartiṣyate* = will occur, will take place

📖 **One mind, having made focus of vision of another mind, the first mind will become aim of other mind, and <u>mix up of minds</u> will occur.**

4.22 चितेरप्रतिसंक्रमायास्तदाकारापत्तौ स्वबुद्धिसंवेदनम् ।

ćitterapratisaṅkramāyāstadākārapattau svabuddhisaṁvedanam

(ćiter-apratisaṅkramāyās-tadākārāpattau sva-buddhi-saṁvedanam)

(i) चितेः *ćiteḥ* = चेतन–शक्तेः, चैतन्यस्य, जीवनस्य शक्तेः, पुरुषस्य of the ātmā

(o) अप्रतिसंक्रमायाः *apratisaṅkramāyāḥ* =

(ii) अप्रति *aprati* = स्वस्य, स्वकं, निज on its own

(iii) संक्रमाया *saṅkramāyāḥ* = सहगमनस्य, वेदनस्य, अनुभूतेः, अभिज्ञातस्य is actionless and unattached

(iv) तथापि *tathāpi* = even then

(o) तदाकारापत्तौ *tadākārāpattau* =

(v) तदाकार *tadākāra* = तद्रूपम्, तन्मयम् like, like that

(vi) आपत्तौ *apattau* = प्राप्तौ, भूत्वा having become

(o) स्व-बुद्धि-संवेदनम् *sva-buddhi-sam̃vedanam* =

(vii) स्व *sva* = स्वस्य, निज own

(viii) बुद्धेः *buddheḥ* = चेतसः, चित्तस्य of mind

(ix) संवेदनं *sam̃vedanam* = ज्ञानम्, प्रतीतिः, अनुभवः, बोधः perceive

(x) भवति *bhavati* = becomes, occurs, happens

📖 **The *ātmā* is actionless and unattached on its own, even then having become like own mind, is able to perceive the mind.**

✍ Comments : *Atma* is actionless and unattached, but is able to receive the mind.

4.23 द्रष्टृदृश्योपरक्तं चित्तं सर्वार्थम् ।

draṣṭṛdṛśyoparaktam ćittam sarvārtham

(draṣṭṛ-dṛśyoparaktam ćittam sarvārtham)

() द्रष्टृ-दृश्य-उपरक्तं *draṣṭṛ-dṛśya-uparaktam* =

(i) द्रष्ट्रा सह *draṣṭṛ sah* = आत्मना सह, पुरुषेण सह, चेतन-शक्तिना सह with ātmā

(ii) दृश्येन *dṛśyena* = वस्तुना, विषयेण सह, चित्रेण सह with a thing, with the object

(iii) उपरक्तं *uparaktam* = रक्तं, सक्तं, ग्रस्तम्, आसक्तं connected

(iv) चित्तम् *ćittam* = चेतः, मनः the mind

(v) सर्व-अर्थम् *sarva-artham* = यथार्थं, उचितम्, युक्तं, सम्यक्, सत्यम् everything feels real

(vi) भवति *bhavati* = is, becomes, occurs, happens

📖 **The mind being connected with *ātmā* and with the object, everything feels real.**

✍ Comments : Mind being connected with the *atma* and the objects, everything is real to it.

4.24 तदसंख्येयवासनाभिश्चित्रमपि परार्थं संहत्यकारित्वात् ।

tadasaṅkhyeyavāsanābhiscittramapi parārtham saṁhatyakāritvāt

(tad-asaṅkhyeya-vāsanābhis-cittram-api parārtham saṁhatya-kāritvāt)

(i) तत् *tat* = तत् चित्तम् that mind

(o) असंख्येय-वासनाभि: *asaṅkhyeya-vāsanābhis* =

(ii) असंख्याभि: *asaṅkhyabhiḥ* = बहुभि:, अनेकाभि:, अगणिताभि:, अगण्याभि: infinite

(iii) वासनाभि: *vāsanābhis* = कामनाभि:, प्रत्याशाभि:, इच्छाभि:, वाञ्छभि: desires

(iv) चित्रम् *cittram* = दृश्यम्, दृष्टम्, प्रतिकृतिम्, छायाम् the object of

(v) अपि = भूत्वा अपि = being also

(vi) पर-अर्थम् *para-artham* = परस्य हेतवे, अन्यस्य प्रयोजनाय for other causes

(vii) सम्-हत्य-कारित्वात् *saṁhatya-kāritvāt* = संमिलित-कर्तृत्वात्, परस्पर-कार्यात् is cooperative

📖 **That mind, being the object of infinite desires, is cooperative for other causes.**

आत्म-भाव-भावना-विनिवृत्ति: ।

ātma-bhāva-bhāvanā-vinivṛttiḥ

87. Selflessness

4.25 विशेषदर्शिन आत्मभावभावनाविनिवृत्ति: ।

viśeṣadarśina ātmabhāvabhāvanāvinivṛttiḥ

(viśeṣa-darśina ātma-bhāva-bhāvanāvinivṛttiḥ)

(o) विशेष-दर्शिनः *viśeṣa-darśinaḥ* =

(i) विशेषं *viśeṣam* = यथार्थं, सत्य-स्वरूपम् real form

(ii) दर्शिनः *darśinaḥ* = पश्यतः beholder of

(iii) योगिनः *yoginaḥ* = of the yogī

(o) आत्म-भाव-भावना-विनिवृत्तिः *ātma-bhāva-bhāvanāvinivṛttiḥ* =

(iv) आत्मनः *ātmanaḥ* = स्वस्य, स्वकीयस्य own self

(v) भावस्य *bhāvasya* = प्रकृतेः, सत्तायाः, विचारस्य, मनोविकारस्य, वृत्तेः knowning about self

(vi) भावनायाः *bhāvanāyāḥ* = विमर्शस्य, विचारस्य, स्मृत्यानुभावजचित्तस्य संस्कारस्य thinking

(vii) विनिवृत्तिः *vinivṛttiḥ* = निवृत्तिः, उपरमः going away, departure

(viii) भवति *bhavati* = becomes, occurs, happens,

📖 Of the *yogī* who is beholder of his own real form, goes away thinking about "knowing who am I, why am I here, what is my purpose, ...etc."

4.26 तदा विवेकनिम्नं कैवल्यप्राग्भारं चित्तम् ।

tadā vivekanimnam kaivalyaprāgbhāram ćittam

(tadā viveka-nimnam kaivalya-prāg-bhāram ćittam)

(i) तदा *tadā* = तदनु, तत् पश्चात्, ततः thereafter, then

(ii) योगिनः *yoginaḥ* = of the yogī

(iii) चित्तम् *ćittam* = हृदयम्, मनः mind

(o) विवेक-निम्नम् *viveka-nimnam* =

(iv) विवेकेन *vivekena* = विचारेण, सदसज्ज्ञानेन having understood the truth about self

(v) निम्नं *nimnam* = नतम्, विनीतम्, अपनीतम् humble

(o) कैवल्य-प्राग्भारम् *kaivalya-prāg-bhāram* =

(vi) कैवल्यस्य प्रति *kaivalyasya prati* = ससंसृष्टतायाः, मोक्षस्य, मुक्तेः, निर्वाणस्य प्रति towards liberation

(vii) प्राग्भारं *prāg-bhāram* = प्रवणम्, प्रणतम्, प्रवर्तितम् inclined

(viii) भवति *bhavati* = is, becomes, occurs, happens

Thereafter, having understood the truth about self (*ātmā*), the mind of the humbled *yogī* becomes inclined towards liberation.

4.27 तच्छिद्रेषु प्रत्ययान्तराणि संस्कारेभ्यः ।

taććhidreṣu pratyāntarāṇi saṁskārebhyaḥ

(tać-ćhidreṣu pratyāntarāṇi saṁskārebhyaḥ)

(i) तत् *tat* = तेषु = in those

(ii) छिद्रेषु *ćhidreṣu* = मनसः व्यवधानेषु, अवकाशेषु, अभ्यन्तरकालेषु, अनरावसरेषु, उपशमेषु, विरामेषु intervening spaces

(iii) संस्कारेभ्यः *saṁskārebhyaḥ* = संस्करणेभ्यः, मानसी–शिक्षाभ्यः, पूर्ववासनाभ्यः, सङ्गप्रभावेभ्यः due to previous impressions

(o) प्रत्यय–अन्तराणि *pratyā-atarāṇi* =

(iv) अन्तराणि *atarāṇi* = अन्यानि, इतराणि, अपराणि other

(v) प्रत्ययाः *pratyāḥ* = विचाराः, कल्पनाः, सङ्कल्पाः, मनोगताः, भावनाः, आभासः thoughts

(vi) आगच्छन्ति *āgaćchanti* = उद्भवन्ति occur

In those intervening spaces other thoughts occur due to <u>previous impressions</u>.

4.28 हानमेषां क्लेशवदुक्तम् ।

hānameṣām kleśavaduktam *(hānam-eṣām kleśavad-uktam)*

(i) एषाम् *eṣām* = एषां संस्काराणां, संस्कार–प्रभवानाम्, मानसी–शिक्षाणाम् of these previous impressions

(ii) हानम् *hānam* = हानिः, क्षयः, विनाशः, ह्रासः the removal

(iii) क्लेशवत् *kleśavat* = दुःखम् इव is like a pain

(iv) उक्तम् अस्ति *uktam asti* = इति उक्तम् it is said that

📖 **It is said that, the removal of these previous impressions is painful.**

समाधिः ।

samādhiḥ

88. Meditation

4.29 प्रसख्यानेऽप्यकुसीदस्य सर्वथा विवेकख्यातेर्धर्ममेघः समाधिः ।

prasakhyāne'pyakusīdasya sarvathā

vivekakhyāterdharmameghaḥ samādhiḥ

(prasakhyāne-'pyakusīdasya sarvathā viveka-khyāter-dharma-meghaḥ samādhiḥ)

(i) प्रसख्याने *prasakhyāne* = आत्मानुसन्धाने, आत्मनिरूपणे, आत्म-अन्वेषणे, आत्म-परिक्षणे on self examination

(ii) अपि *api* = also

(iii) यस्य योगिनः *yasya yoginaḥ* = of the yogī whose

(iv) विश्वासः *viśvāsaḥ* = faith

(v) अकुसीदस्य *akusīdasya* = च्युतः, पतितः, स्रस्तः, अदृढः, विगलितः dwindled

(vi) अस्ति *asti* = is

(vii) तस्य अपि *tasya api* = even his

(viii) सर्वथा *sarvathā* = सामस्त्येन, सर्व-प्रकारेण in every which way

(o) विवेक-ख्यातेः *viveka-khyāteḥ* =

(ix) विवेकस्य *vivekasya* = विचारस्य, सदसज्ज्ञानस्य, सत्यज्ञानस्य of knowing the truth

(x) ख्यातेः *khyāteḥ* = कीर्तेः, प्रभावस्य being powerful

(xi) धर्म-मेघ-समाधिः *dharma-meghaḥ samādhiḥ* = "धर्ममेघ" समाधिः 'dharmamegha' samādhiḥ

(xii) भवति *bhavati* = is, becomes, occurs, happens

📖 **On self examination of the *yogī* whose faith has dwindled, even his will of knowing the truth being powerful in every which way, *'dharmamegha' samādhiḥ* occurs.**

4.30 ततः क्लेशकर्मनिवृत्तिः ।

tataḥ kleśakarmanivṛttiḥ *(tataḥ kleśa-karma-nivṛttiḥ)*

(i) ततः *tataḥ* = तस्याः समाध्याः योगेन with the help of that samādhiḥ

(o) क्लेश-कर्म-निवृत्तिः *kleśa-karma-nivṛttiḥ* =

(ii) क्लेशस्य *kleśasya* = दुःखानाम्, पीडानाम् of pains

(iii) कर्म च *karma cha* = कर्माणाम्, कृत्यानाम् and of karmas

(iv) निवृत्तिः *nivṛttiḥ* = अपचयः, उपरमः, ह्रासः, विरतिः departure

(v) भवति *bhavati* = becomes, occurs, happens

📖 **With the help of that *dharma-megha samādhiḥ,* occurs departure of pains and of *karmas.***

4.31 तदा सर्वावरणमलापेतस्य ज्ञानस्यानन्त्याज्ज्ञेयमल्पम् ।

tadā sarvāvaraṇamalāpetasya jñānasyānantyājjñeyamalpam

(tadā sarvāvaraṇa-malāpetasya jñānasyānantyāj-jñeyam-alpam)

(i) तदा *tadā* = तस्मिन् काले at that time

(o) सर्व-आवरण-मल-अपेतस्य *sarvāvaraṇa-mala-apetasya* =

(ii) सर्वस्य *sarva* = सकलस्य, समस्तस्यम्, अशेषस्य, निःशेषस्य of all

(iii) मलस्य *malasya* = अवकरस्य, कल्कस्य, अपकरस्य impurities

(iv) आवरणं *āvaraṇam* = आच्छदनम्, मेघ:, पुट: the covering of, blanket of

(v) अपेतस्य *apetasya* = गतस्य, निर्गतस्य, निर्धूतस्य removed

(vi) ज्ञानस्य *jñānasy* = बोधस्य, प्रतीते: of understanding

(vii) आनन्त्यात् *ānantyāt* = वैपुल्यात्, नि:सीमाया: as a result of infinity

(viii) ज्ञेयम् *jñeyam* = ज्ञातव्यम् what is ought to be known

(ix) अल्पम् *alpam* = लघु विद्यते becomes sparse

📖 **At that time, the blanket of all impurities being removed, and as a result of infinity of understanding, what is ought to be known becomes sparse.**

✍ Comments : when the blanket of impurities of previous impressions is removed, nothing remains to be known.

4.32 तत: कृतार्थानां परिणामक्रमसमाप्तिर्गुणानाम् ।

tataḥ kṛtārthānām pariṇāmakramasamāpatirguṇānām

(tataḥ kṛtārthānām pariṇāma-krama-samāpatir-guṇānām)

(i) तत: *tataḥ* = यदा ज्ञेयं अल्पं विद्यते तदा when what is ought to be known becomes sparse

(ii) कृतार्थानाम् *kṛtārthānām* = पूर्णकामानां, कृतकार्यानाम् accomplishments

(iii) गुणानाम् *guṇānām* = धर्माणां, स्वभावानाम्, प्रकृतीनाम् their nature

(o) परिणाम-क्रम-समाप्ति: *pariṇāma-krama-samāpattiḥ* =

(iv) तेषां सिद्धीनां परिणामानां *teṣām siddhīnām pariṇāmān* = फलानाम्, अनुषङ्गानाम्, निर्गमानाम्, फलितार्थानाम्, प्रत्ययानाम् and their successes, fruits

(v) समप्ति: *samāpatiḥ* = अन्त:, अवसानम्, निवृत्ति: departure, end

(vi) भवति *bhavati* = occurs

📖 **When what is ought to be known becomes sparse, the fruits of accomplishments, their nature and their successes come to an end.**

✍ Comments : When nothing remains to be known, the fruits of accomplishments come to an end.

क्रमः ।

kramaḥ

89. Sequential Perception

4.33 क्षणप्रतियोगी परिणामापरान्तनिर्ग्राह्यः क्रमः ।

kṣaṇapratiyogī pariṇāmāparāntanirgrāhyaḥ kramaḥ

(kṣaṇa-pratiyogī pariṇāmāparānta-nir-grāhyaḥ kramaḥ)

(o) क्षण-प्रतियोगी *kṣaṇa-pratiyogī* =

(i) प्रतिक्षणं *pratikṣaṇam* = प्रतिनिमेशम् at each moment sequentially

(ii) परिवर्ती *parivartī* = विकारी a transient, impermanent

(iii) पदार्थः *padārthaḥ* = वस्तु thing

(o) परिणाम-अपरान्त-निर्ग्राह्यः *pariṇāmāparānta-nir-grāhyaḥ* =

(iv) यस्य *yasya* = of which

(v) स्वरूपं *svarupam* = स्वभावः, गुणः, धर्मः, प्रकृतिः nature

(vi) परिणामस्य *pariṇāmasya* = फलस्य of fruit

(vii) अपरान्तं *aparāntam* = अनन्तरम् at the end

(viii) निर्ग्राह्यः *nir-grāhyaḥ* = दृश्यते, स्पष्टं भवति becomes clear

(ix) सः *saḥ* = that

(x) विधिः *vidhiḥ* = नियमः process

(xi) 'क्रमः' *'kramaḥ,'* = sequential perception

(xii) इति उच्यते *iti uchyate* = is known as, is called as

📖 **At each moment sequentially, a transient thing, of which nature of fruit becomes clear at the end, that process is called as *'kramaḥ,'* (sequential** perception).

✍ Comments : *Krarma* is that sequential process by which nature of fruit becomes clear. Remember, *karma* is different than *krama*.

कैवल्यम् ।

kaivalyam

90. Finl liberation

4.34 पुरुषार्थशून्यानां गुणानां प्रतिप्रसवः कैवल्यं स्वरूपप्रतिष्ठा वा चितिशक्तेरिति ।

puruṣārthasūnyānām guṇānām pratiprasavaḥ kaivalyam svarūpapratiṣṭhā vā ćitiśakteriti

(puruṣārtha-sūnyānām guṇānām pratiprasavaḥ kaivalyam svarūpa-pratiṣṭhā vā ćiti-śakter-iti)

(o) पुरुषार्थ-शून्यानाम् *puruṣārtha-sūnyānām* =

(i) पुरुषार्था: *puruṣārthāḥ* = धर्मार्थकाममोक्षा:, चतुर्-पुरुष-प्रयोजनानि the four basic stages of human life

(ii) शून्यानां *sūnyānām* = विहीनानाम्, रहितानाम् those who have completed and come to a zero state

(iii) गुणानाम् *guṇānām* = वृत्तीनाम् of their guṇas

(iv) प्रतिप्रसवः *pratiprasavaḥ* = अपवादस्य अपवादः, विशेषेणस्य आवर्तनम् return to original state

(v) 'कैवल्यम्' *'kaivalyam,'* = liberation

(vi) अस्ति *asti* = is

(vii) वा *vā* = or

(viii) चितिशक्तेः *ćiti-śakteḥ* = प्रभावस्य, सामर्थ्यस्य, तेजसः, ओजसः, ऊर्जस्य, सत्तायाः, मायायाः of the sway of the ātmā

(o) स्वरूप-प्रतिष्ठा *svarūpa-pratiṣṭhā* =

(ix) स्वरूपस्य *svarūpa* = रूपस्य, प्रकृतेः to its original point

(x) प्रतिष्ठा *pratiṣṭhā* = गौरव:, स्थापना return

(xi) अस्ति *asti* = is

(xii) इति मन्तव्यम् *iti mantavyam* = thus one should understand.

Those who have completed the four basic stages of human life and come to a zero state, return of their *guṇas* to original state is *'kaivalyam'* (liberation), or return of the sway of the *ātmā* to its original point, is *(kaivalya)* thus one should understand.

Comments : He who has completed the four stages of the *vaidic* life, his life comes to zero state and returns to original state. That original point is *kaivalya*.

APPENDIX

English Alphabetical Index to the Yoga Sūtras

A

abhāva-pratyayālambanā vṛttir-nidrā 1.10

abhyāsa-vairāgyābhyām tan-nirodhaḥ 1.12

ahiṁsāsatyāsteya-brahmacharyāparigrahāḥ- 2.30

ahimsāpratiṣṭhāyām tat-sannidhau vaira-tyāgaḥ 2.35

anityāśuchi-duḥkhānātmasu nitya-śuci- 2.5

anubhūta-viṣayāsampramoṣaḥ smṛtiḥ 1.11

aparigraha-sthairyam janma-kathanta- 2.39

asteya-pratiṣṭhāyam sarva-ratno-pasthānam 2.37

atītānāgatam svarūpato'styadhva-bhedad- 4.12

atha yogānuśāsanam 1.1

avidyā kṣetram-uttareṣām prasupta-tanu- 2.4

avidyāsmitārāga-dveṣābhiniveśāḥ kleśāḥ 2.3

B

bāhyābhyantara-stambha-vṛttir-deśa-kāla- 2.50

bāhyābhyantara-viṣayākṣepī ćturthaḥ 2.51

baleṣu hasti-balādīni 3.24

bandha-kāraṇa-śaithilyāt-praćāra-saṁvedanāć- 3.38

bhavapratyayo videha-prakṛti-layānām 1.19

bhir-kalpitā vṛttir-mahāvidehā tatah- 3.43

bhuvana-jñānam sūrye saṁyamāt 3.26

brahmaćarya-pratiṣṭhāyam vīrya-lābhaḥ 2.38

C

ćandre tārāvyūha-jñānam 3.27

ćittāntara-dṛśye buddhi-buddher- 4.21

ćitter-apratisaṅkramāyās-tadākārapattau- 4.22

D

deśa-bandha-śćittasya dhāraṇā 3.1

dharaṇāsu- ća yogyatā manasaḥ 2.53

dhruve tad-gati-jñānam 3.28

dhyāna-heyāstad-vṛttayaḥ 2.11

dṛg-darśana-śaktyo-'rekātmatevāsmitā 2.6

dṛṣṭānuśrāvika-viṣaya-vitṛṇasya vaśikāra- 4.1

K

āyāākāśayoḥ sambandha-saṁyamal-laghu-tūla- 3.42

kāya-rūpa-saṁyamāt-tat-grāhya-śakti- 3.21

kāye-ndriya-siddhir-śuddhi-kṣayāt-tapasaḥ 2.43

kaṇtha-kūpe kṣut-pipāsa-nivṛttiḥ 3.30

karmāśuklākṛṣṇam yoginas-tri-vidham-itareṣām 4.7

kleśa-karma-vipākāśayair-aprāmarṣṭaḥ puruṣa- 1.24

kleśa-mūlaḥ karmāśayo dṛṣṭādṛṣṭa-janma- 2.12

kṛtārtham prati naṣṭam-apyanaṣṭam tadnya- 2.22

kramānyatvam pariṇamānyatvam hetuḥ 3.15

kṣīṇa-vṛtter-abhijātasy-eva maṇer-grahitṛ- 1.41

kṣaṇa-pratiyogī pariṇāmāparānta-nir- 4.33

kṣaṇa-tat-kramayoḥ saṁyamād-vivekajam- 3.52

kūrma-nāḍyām sthairyam 3.31

M

aitrī-karuṇāmudito-pekṣaṇām sukha-du:kha- 1.33

maitryādiṣu balāni 3.23

mṛdu-madhya-adhimātratvaat-tatao-'pi viśeṣaḥ 1.22

mūrdh-jyotiṣi siddha-darśanam 3.32

N

a ća tat- sālambanam tasyāviṣayaī-bhūtatvāt 3.20

na ćaika-ćitta-tantram vastu tad-pramāṇakam- 4.16

na tat-svābhāsam dṛśyatvāt 4.19

nābhi-ćakre kāya-vyūha-jñānam 3.29

nimittam-aprayojakam prakṛtinān varaṇa- 4.3

nirmāṇa-chittānyasmitāmātrāt 4.4

nir-vićāra-vaiśāradye-'dhyātma-prasādaḥ 1.47

tad-artha eva dṛśyasyātmā 2.21
tad-asaṅkhyeya-vāsanābhis-ćittram-api - 4.24
tad-evā̃-rtha-mātra-nirbhāsam svarūpa- 3.3
tad-vairāgyād-api doṣa-bīja-kṣaye kaivalyam 3.50
taj-jaḥ saṁskāro-ʻanya-saṁskāra-pratibandhī 1.50
ta-jjapas-tadartha-bhāvanam 1.28
taj-jayāt-prajñālokaḥ 3.5
tapaḥ svādhyāye-śvara-praṇidhāni kriyāyogaḥ 2.1
tasmin-sati śsāsa-praśvāsayor-gati-vićchedaḥ- 2.49
tasya bhūmiṣu viniyogaḥ 3.6
tasya hetur-avidyā 2.24
tasya praśāntavāhitā saṁskārāt 3.10
tasya vāćakaḥ praṇavaḥ 1.27
tasyāpi nirodhe sarva-nirodhānnir-bījaḥ- 1.51
tasyasaptadhā prānta-bhūmiḥ prajñā 2.27
tataḥ kṛtārthānām pariṇāma-krama-samāpattir- 4.32
tataḥ kṣīyate prakāṣāvaraṇam 2.52
tataḥ lkeśa-karma-nivṛttiḥ 4.30
tataḥ manojavitvam vikaraṇa-bhāvaḥ pradhāna- 3.48
tataḥ paramā vaśyatendryāṇām 2.55
tataḥ prātibha-śrāvaṇa-vedanādarśāsvāda- 3.36
tataḥ pratyak-ćetanādhigamo-ʻpya-ntarāyābhā- 1.29
tataḥ punaḥ śānto-ditau tulya-pratyayau - 3.12
tatas-tad-vipākānuguṇānām-evābhivyaktir- 4.8
tato dvandvā̃-nabhighātaḥ 2.48
tato-ʻṇimādi-prādurbhāvaḥ - 3.45
tat-param puruṣa-khyāter-guṇa-vaitṛṣṇyam 1.16
tat-pratiṣedhārtham-eka-tattvābhyāsaḥ 1.32
tatra dhyānajam-anāśayam 4.6
tatra nir-atiśatam sarva-bījam 1.25
tatra pratyai-ktānatā dhyānam 3.2
tatra śabdārtha-jñāna-vikalpaiḥ saṅkīrṇā - 1.42
tatra sthitau yatno-ʻbhyāsaḥ 1.13
te lhāda-paritāpa-falāḥ puṇyāpuṇya-hetutvāt 2.14
te prati-prasava-heyāḥ sūkṣmāḥ 2.10
te samādhāvupasargāḥ vyutthāne siddhataḥ 3.37
te vyakta-sūkṣmā guṇātmanaḥ 4.13
trayam-antaraṅgam pūrvebhyaḥ 3.7
trayam-ekatram saṁyamaḥ 3.4

U

udāna-jayāj-jala-paṅka-kaṇṭakādiṣva-saṅg- 3.39

V

vīta-rāga-viṣayam vā ćittam 1.37
vastu-sāmye chitta-bhedāt-tayor-vibhaktaḥ- 4.15
viparyayo mithyājñānam-a-tadrūpa-pratiṣṭham 1.8
virāma-pratyayābhyāsa-pūrvaḥ saṁskāra-śeṣo- 1.18
viśeṣāviśeṣa-linga-mātrālingāni guṇa-parvāṇi 2.19
viśeṣa-darśina ātma-bhāva-bhāvanāvinivṛttiḥ 4.25
viśokā vā jyotiṣmati 1.36
viṣayavatī vā pravṛtti-rutpannā manasaḥ sthiti- 1.35
vitarkā hiṁsādayaḥ kṛta-kāritāanumoditā - 2.34
vitarka-bādhane prati-pakṣa-bhāvanam 2.33
vitarka-vićārānandāsmitānugāmāt- 1.17
viveka-khyātir-aviplavā hanopāyaḥ 2.26
vṛttayaḥ pañća-tayyaḥ kilṣṭākliṣṭāḥ 1.5
vṛtti-sārūpyam-itartra 1.4
vyādhi-styāna-saṁśaya-pramād-ālasyāvirati- 1.30
vyutthāna-nirodha-saṁskārayor-abhibhava- 3.9

Y

yadā dṛṣṭuḥ sva-rūpe-ʻvasthānam 1.3
yama-niyamāsana-prāṇāyāma-partyāhāra- 2.29
yathābhimata-dhyānād-vā 1.39
yogāṅgānuṣṭhānād-aśuddhi-kṣaye- 2.28
yogaś-ćitta-vṛtti-nirodhaḥ 1.2

Sanskrit Alphabetical Index to the Yoga Sūtras

द्रष्टा दृशिमात्रः शुद्धोऽपि प्रत्ययानुपश्यः । 2.20
द्रष्टृदृश्ययोः संयोगो हेयहेतुः । 2.17
द्रष्टुदृश्योपरक्तं चित्तं सर्वार्थम् । 4.23
धारणासु च योग्यता मनसः । 2.53
ध्यानहेयास्तद्वृत्तयः । 2.11
ध्रुवे तद्गतिज्ञानम् । 3.28
न च तत्सालम्बनं तस्याविषयीभूतत्वात् । 3.20
न चैकचित्ततन्त्रं वस्तु तदप्रमाणकं तदा किं स्यात् । 4.16
न तत्स्वाभासं दृश्यत्वात् । 4.19
नाभिचक्रे कायव्यूहज्ञानम् । 3.29
निमित्तमप्रयोजकं प्रकृतीनां वरणभेदस्तु ततः क्षेत्रिकवत् । 4.3
निर्माणचित्तान्यस्मितामात्रात् । 4.4
निर्विचारवैशारद्येऽध्यात्मप्रसादः । 1.47
परमाणुपरममहत्त्वान्तोऽस्य वशीकारः । 1.40
परिणामतापसंस्कारदुःखैर्गुणवृत्तिविरोधाच्च दुःखमेव सर्वं विवेकिनः । 2.15
परिणामत्रयसंयमादतीतानागतज्ञानम् । 3.16
परिणामैकत्वाद्वस्तुतत्त्वम् । 4.14
पुरुषार्थशून्यानां गुणानां प्रतिप्रसवः कैवल्यं - 4.34
पूर्वेषामपि गुरुः कालेनानवच्छेदात् । 1.26
प्रकाशक्रियास्थितिशीलं भूतेन्द्रियात्मकं भोगापवर्गार्थं दृश्यम् । 2.18
प्रच्छर्दन-विधारणाभ्यां वा प्राणस्य । 1.34
प्रातिभाद्वा सर्वम् । 3.33
प्रत्यक्षानुमानागमाः प्रमाणानि । 1.7
प्रत्ययस्य परचित्तज्ञानम् । 3.19
प्रमाणविपर्ययविकल्पनिद्रास्मृतयः । 1.6
प्रयत्नशैथिल्यानन्तसमापत्तिभ्याम् । 2.47
प्रवृत्तिभेदे प्रयोजकं चित्तमेकमनेकेषाम् । 4.5
प्रवृत्त्यालोकन्यासात्सूक्ष्मव्यवहितविप्रकृष्टज्ञानम् । 3.25
प्रसख्यानेऽप्यकुसीदस्य सर्वथा विवेकख्यातेर्धर्ममेघः समाधिः । 4.29
बन्धकारणशैथिल्यात्प्रचारसंवेदनाच्च चित्तस्य परशरीरावेशः । 3.38
बलेषु हस्तिबलादीनि । 3.24
बाह्याभ्यन्तरविषयाक्षेपी चतुर्थः । 2.51
बाह्याभ्यन्तरस्तम्भवृत्तिर्देशकालसंख्याभिः परिदृष्टो दीर्घसूक्ष्मः । 2.50
बहिरकल्पिता वृत्तिर्महाविदेहा ततः प्रकाशावरणक्षयः । 3.43
ब्रह्मचर्यप्रतिष्ठायां वीर्यलाभः । 2.38
भवप्रत्ययो विदेहप्रकृतिलयानाम् । 1.19
भुवनज्ञानं सूर्ये संयमात् । 3.26
मूर्धज्योतिषि सिद्धदर्शनम् । 3.32
मैत्रीकरुणामुदितोपेक्षाणां सुखदुःखपुण्यापुण्यविषयाणा - 1.33
मैत्र्यादिषु बलानि । 3.23
यदा द्रष्टुः स्वरूपेऽवस्थानम् । 1.3
यथाभिमतध्यानाद्वा । 1.39
यमनियमासनप्राणायामप्रत्याहारधारणाध्यानसमाधयोऽष्टावङ्गानि । 2.29
योगश्चित्तवृत्तिनिरोधः । 1.2
योगाङ्गानुष्ठानादशुद्धिक्षये ज्ञानदीप्तिराविवेकख्यातेः । 2.28
रूपलावण्यबलवज्रसंहननत्वानि कायसम्पत् । 3.46
वस्तुसाम्ये चित्तभेदात्तयोर्विभक्तः पन्थाः । 4.15
विशोका वा ज्योतिष्मती । 1.36
विशेषाविशेषलिङ्गमात्रालिङ्गानि गुणपर्वाणि । 2.19
विशेषदर्शिन आत्मभावभावनाविनिवृत्तिः । 4.25
विपर्ययो मिथ्याज्ञानमतद्रूपप्रतिष्ठम् । 1.8
विषयवती वा प्रवृत्तिरुत्पन्ना मनसः स्थितिनिबन्धनी । 1.35
वितर्कबाधने प्रतिपक्षभावनम् । 2.33
वितर्कविचारानन्दास्मितानुगमात्सम्प्रज्ञातः । 1.17
वितर्का हिंसादयः कृतकारिताअनुमोदिता लोभक्रोधमोहपूर्वका - 2.34
विरामप्रत्ययाभ्यासपूर्वः संस्कारशेषोऽन्यः । 1.18
विवेकख्यातिरविप्लवा हानोपायः । 2.26
वीतरागविषयं वा चित्तम् । 1.37
वृत्तिसारूप्यमितरत्र । 1.4
वृत्तयः पञ्चतय्यः क्लिष्टाक्लिष्टाः । 1.5
व्याधिस्त्यानसंशयप्रमादालस्याविरतिभ्रान्तिदर्शनालब्धभूमि - 1.30
व्युत्थाननिरोधसंस्कारयोरभिभवप्रादुर्भावौ - 3.9
शब्दज्ञानानुपाती वस्तुशून्यो विकल्पः । 1.9
शब्दार्थप्रत्ययानामितरेतराध्यासात्सङ्करस्तत्प्रविभागसंयमात्सर्वभूत - 3.17
शान्तोदिताव्यपदेश्यधर्मानुपाति धर्मी । 3.14
शौचसन्तोषतपःस्वाध्यायेश्वरप्रणिधानि नियमाः । 2.32
शौचात्स्वाङ्गजुगुप्सा परैरसंसर्गः । 2.40
श्रद्धावीर्यस्मृतिसमाधिप्रज्ञापूर्वक इतरेषाम् । 1.20
श्रुतानुमानप्रज्ञाभ्यामन्यविषया विशेषार्थात् । 1.49
श्रोत्राकाशयोः सम्बन्धसंयमाद्दिव्यं श्रोत्रम् । 3.41
स तु दीर्घकालनैरन्तर्यसत्काराऽऽसेवितो दृढभूमिः । 1.14
संस्कारसाक्षात्करणात्पूर्वजातिज्ञानम् । 3.18
सति मूले तद्विपाको जात्यायुर्भोगाः । 2.13
सदा ज्ञाताश्चित्तवृत्तयस्तत्प्रभोः पुरुषस्यापरिणामित्वात् । 4.18
सन्तोषादनुत्तमसुखलाभः । 2.42
समाधिभावनार्थः क्लेशतनूकरणार्थश्च । 2.2
समाधिसिद्धिरीश्वरप्रणिधानात् । 2.45
समानजयाज्ज्वलनम् । 3.40
सत्त्वपुरुषयोरत्यन्तासङ्कीर्णयोः प्रत्ययाविशेषो भोगः - 3.35
सत्त्वपुरुषयोः शुद्धिसाम्ये कैवल्यम् । 3.55
सत्त्वपुरुषान्यताख्यातिमात्रस्य सर्वभावाधिष्ठातृत्वं सर्व-ज्ञातृत्वमं च । 3.49
सत्त्वशुद्धिसौमनस्यएकाग्रेन्द्रियजयाआत्मदर्शनयोग्यत्वानि । 2.41
सत्यप्रतिष्ठायां क्रियाफलाश्रयत्वम् । 2.36
सर्वार्थतैकाग्रतयोः क्षयोदयौ चित्तस्य समाधिपरिणामः । 3.11
सुखानुशयी रागः । 2.7
सूक्ष्मविषयत्वं चालिङ्गपर्यवसानम् । 1.45
सोपक्रमं निरूपक्रमं च कर्म तत्संयमादपरान्तज्ञानमरिष्टेभ्यो वा । 3.22
स्थान्युपनिमन्त्रेण सङ्गस्मयाकरणं पुनरनिष्टप्रसङ्गात् । 3.51
स्थिरसुखमासनम् । 2.46
स्थूलस्वरूपसूक्ष्मान्वयार्थवत्त्वसंयमाद्भूतजयः । 3.44
स्मृतिपरिशुद्धौ स्वरूपशून्येवार्थमात्रनिर्भासा निर्वितर्का । 1.43
स्वप्ननिद्राज्ञानालम्बनं वा । 1.38
स्वरसवाही विदुषोऽपि तथारूढोऽभिनिवेशः । 2.9
स्वविषयसम्प्रयोगे चित्तस्वरूपानुकार इवेन्द्रियाणां प्रत्याहारः । 2.54
स्वस्वामिशक्त्योः स्वरूपोपलब्धिहेतुः संयोगः । 2.23
स्वाध्यायादिष्टदेवतासम्प्रयोगः । 2.44
हानमेषां क्लेशवदुक्तम् । 4.28
हृदये चित्तसंवित् । 3.34
हेतुफलाश्रयालम्बनैः संगृहीतत्वादेषामभावे तदभावः । 4.11
हेयं दुःखमनागतम् । 2.16

SIXTY MOST COMMON ASANAS

ॐ ह्राम् ह्रीम् ह्रूम् ह्रैम् ह्रोम् ।

मित्ररविसूर्यभानुखगपूषहिरण्यगर्भमरीच्यादित्यसवित्रार्कभास्करेभ्यो नमो नमः । ।

1. *Adhomukha-śvānāsana* अधोमुखश्वानासन *(adhomukh = face down, śvān = dog)*
2. *Ardha-matsyāsana* अर्धमत्स्यासन *(ardha = half, matsya = fish)*
3. *Ardha-padmāsana* अर्धपद्मासन *(ardha = half, padma = lotus)*
4. *Baddha-koṇāsana* बद्धकोणासन *(baddha = restrained, koṇa = angle)*
5. *Baddha-psdmāsana* बद्धपद्मासन *(baddha = restricted, padma = lotus)*
6. *Bakāsana* बकासन *(bak = stork)*
7. *Bhāradvājāsana* भरद्वाजासन *(bhāradvāj = sky-lark)*
8. *Bhadrāsana* भद्रासन *(bhadra = Shiva)*
9. *Bhujaṅgāsana* भुजंगासन *(bhujaṅga = snake)*
10. *Ćakrāsana* चक्रासन *(chakra = wheel)*
11. *Danḍāsana* दंडासन *(daṇḍa = rod, stick)*
12. *Dhanurāsana* धनुरासन *(Dhanur = bow)*
13. *Gomukhāsana* गोमुखासन *(gomukha = face of a cow)*
14. *Gorakṣaṇāsana* गोरक्षणासन *(gorakṣaṇa = cow)*
15. *Halāsana* हलासन *(hal = plough)*
16. *Jānuśīrṣāsana* जानुशीर्षासन *(jānu = knee, śīrṣa= head)*
17. *Karṇapīḍāsana* कर्णपीडासन *(karṇa = ear, pīḍā = pain)*
18. *Kukkuṭāsana* कुक्कुटासन *(kukkuṭa = hen, rooster)*
19. *Makarāsana* मकरासन *(makara = alligator)*
20. *Manḍukāsana* मण्डुकासन *(maṇḍuka = frog)*
21. *Marhārāsana* मार्जारासन *(mārjāra = cat)*
22. *Marichyāsana* मरीच्यासन *(marichi = a ray of light, sun)*
23. *Matsyāsana* मत्स्यासन *(matsya = fish)*
24. *Mayūrāsana* मयूरासन *(mayūra = peacock)*
25. *Mūlabandhāsana* मूलबन्धासन *(mūla = root, bandha = binding)*
26. *Muktāsana* मुक्तासन *(mukta = free, natural,,uninhibited)*
27. *Naukāsana* नौकासन *(naukā = boat)*
28. *Pād-paśćimottānāsana* पादपश्चिमोत्तानासन *(pad = legs, feet, paśćima = back side of the body, uttāna = raising)*
29. *Padmāsana* पद्मासम *(padma = lotus)*
30. *Padma-mayūrāsana* पद्ममयूरासन *(padma = lotus, mayūra = peacock)*
31. *Padottānāsana* पदोत्तानासन *(pād = feet, uttāna = lifting up)*
32. *Parvatāsana* पर्वतासन *(parvata = mountain)*
33. *Paśćimottānāsana* पश्चिमोत्तानासन *(paśćima = back of the body, uttāna = lifting up)*
34. *Pavanamuktāsana* पवनमुक्तासन *(pavana = wind, mukta = releave)*
35. *Prasārit-pādottānāsana* प्रसारितपादोत्तानासन *(prasārita = spread, pād = legs, uttana = raising up)*
36. *Sīrṣāsana* शीर्षासन *(śīrṣa = head)*
37. *Śalabhāsana* शलभासन *(śalabh = grass-hopper, locust)*
38. *Śaśāṅkāsana* शशांकासन *(śaśāṅk = moon)*
39. *Śavāsana* शवासन *(śava = dead body)*
40. *Sarvāṅgāsana* सर्वांगासन *(sarva = whole, aṅga = body)*
41. *Setubandha-sarvāṅgāsana* सेतुबंधसर्वांगासन *(setu = bridge)*
42. *Siddhāsana* सिद्धासन *(siddha = yogī)*
43. *Siṁhāsana* सिंहासन *(siṁha = lion)*
44. *Sukhāsana* सुखासन *(sukha = unbound)*
45. *Supta-Vīrāsana* सुप्तवीरासन *(supta = lying down, vīra = warrior)*
46. *Svastikāsana* स्वस्तिकासन *(svastika = a crossing)*
47. *Taḍāsana* ताडासन *(tāḍa = palm tree)*
48. *Tolāṅgulāsana* तोलांगुलासन *(tola = balance, aṅgula = toes)*
49. *Trikoṇāsana* त्रिकोणासन *(trikoṇa = triangle)*
50. *Urdhva-sarvāṅgāsan* ऊर्ध्वसर्वांगासन *(ūrdhva = up)*
51. *Uṣṭrāsana* उष्ट्रासन *(uṣṭra = camel)*
52. *Utkaṭāsana* उत्कटासन *(utkaṭa = powerful)*
53. *Uttānāsana* उत्तानासन *(uttān = stretched, spread)*
54. *Uttāna-kūrmāsana* उत्तानकूर्मासन *(uttāna = stretched, kurma = turtle)*
55. *Vīrāsana* वीरासन *(vīra = warrior, hero)*
56. *Vajrāsana* वज्रासन *(vajra = thunderbolt)*
57. *Vakrāsana* वक्रासन *(vakra = arched)*
58. *Viparītāsana* विपरीतासन *(viparīta = flipping the body)*
59. *Vṛkṣāsana* वृक्षासन *(vṛkṣa = tree)*
60. *Yogīmudrāsana* योगीमुद्रासन *(mudrā = image, seal, impression)*

BOOKS by Prof. RATNAKAR NARALE

www.ratnakar-books.com

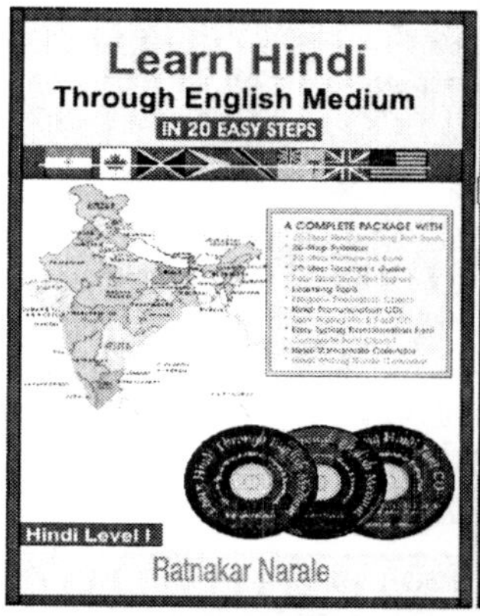

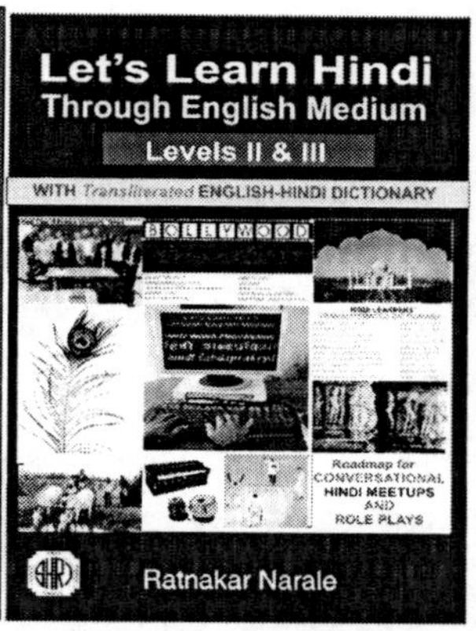

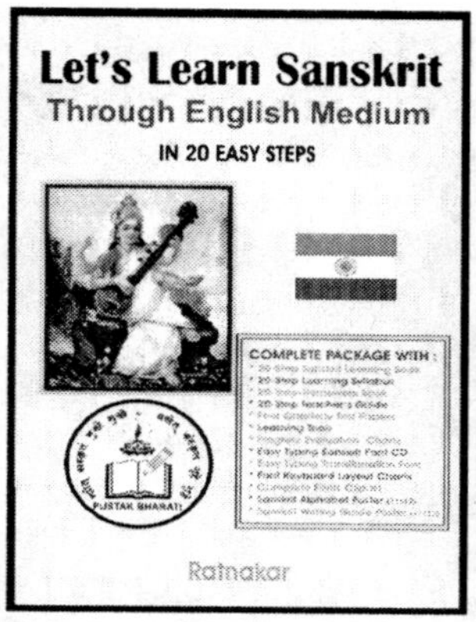

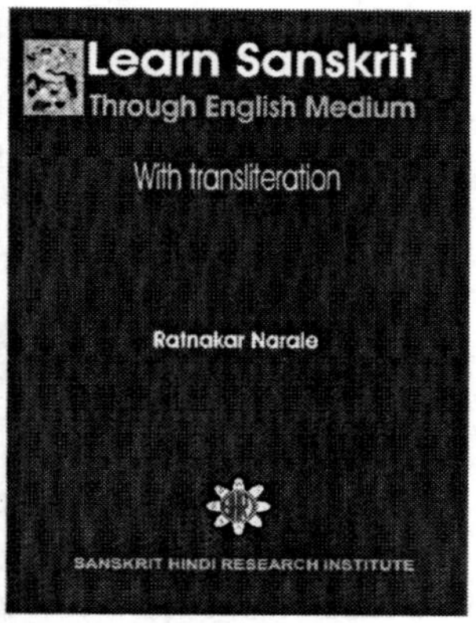

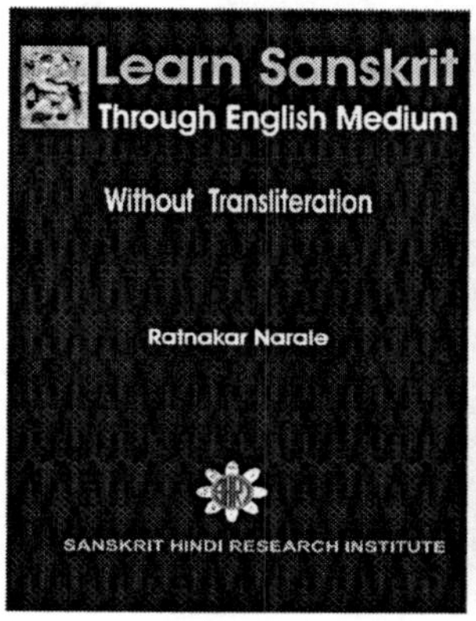

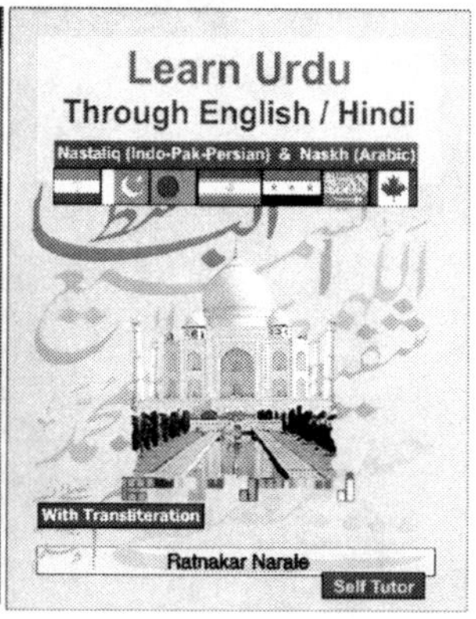

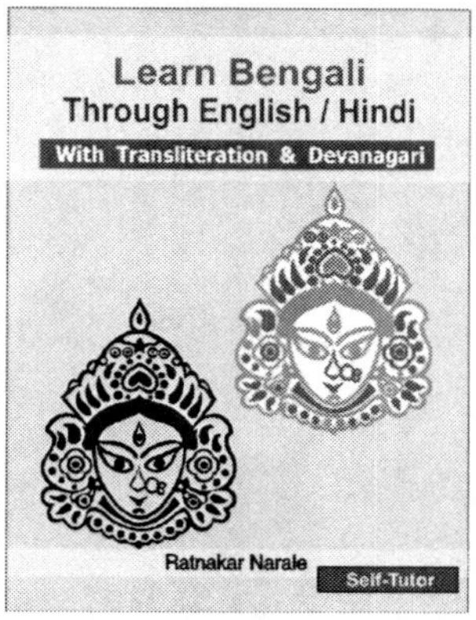

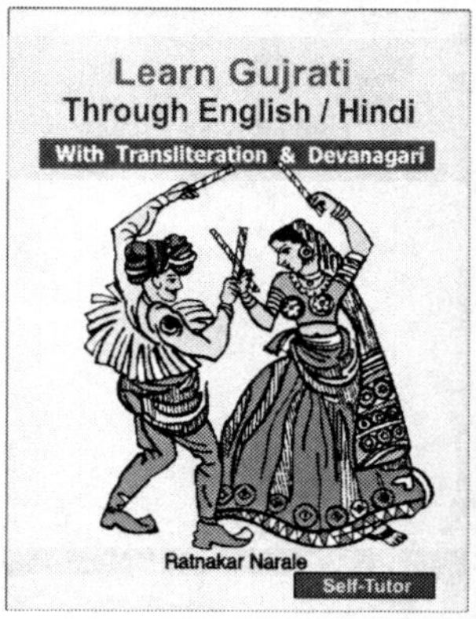

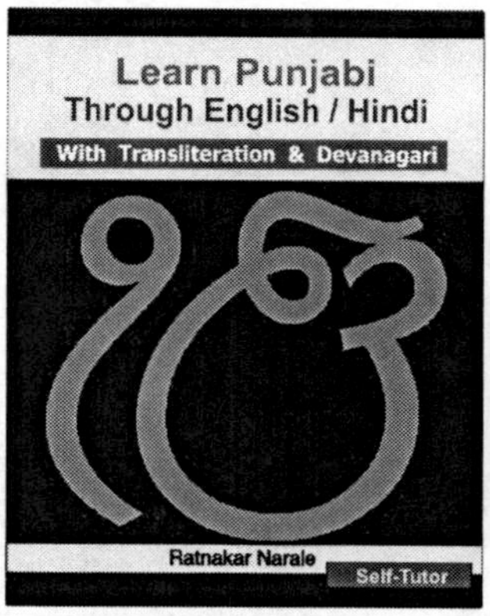

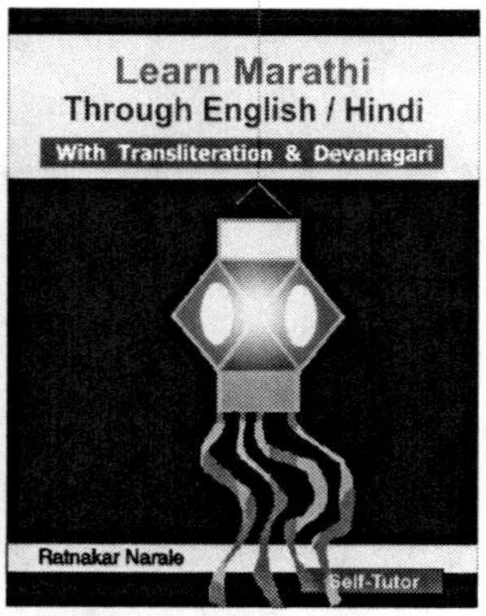

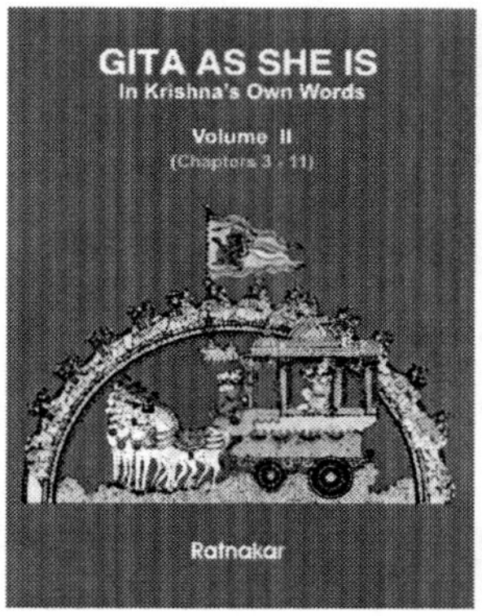

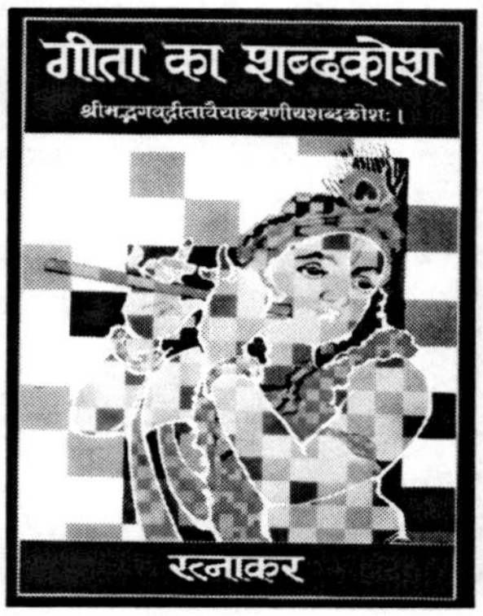

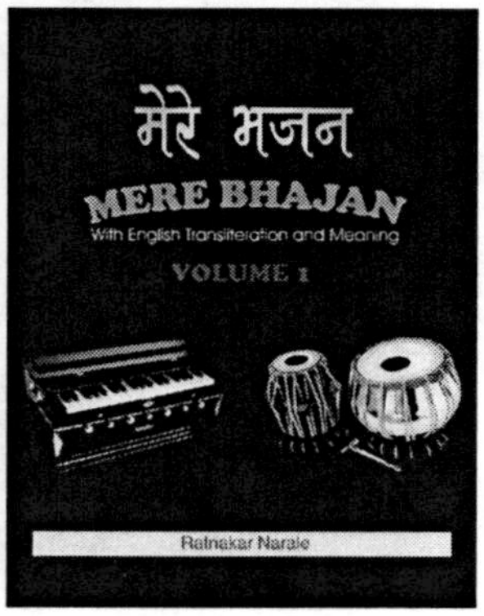

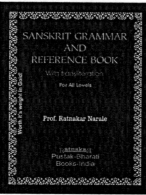

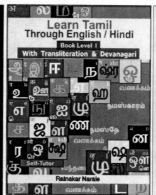

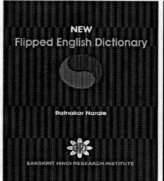

CPSIA information can be obtained at www.ICGtesting.com
Printed in the USA
BVOW04s1025180814
363275BV00030B/1136/P

9 781897 416532